MAKING DISEASE, MAKING CITIZENS

Making Disease, Making Citizens
The Politics of Hepatitis C

SUZANNE FRASER AND KATE SEEAR
Monash University, Australia

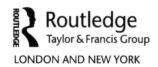

Routledge
Taylor & Francis Group

LONDON AND NEW YORK

First published 2011 by Ashgate Publishing

2 Park Square, Milton Park, Abingdon, Oxon OX14 4RN
711 Third Avenue, New York, NY 10017, USA

Routledge is an imprint of the Taylor & Francis Group, an informa business

First issued in paperback 2016

British Library Cataloguing in Publication Data
Fraser, Suzanne, 1967-
 Making disease, making citizens : the politics of hepatitis C.
 1. Hepatitis C--Social aspects. 2. Hepatitis C--Patients.
 3. Hepatitis C--Treatment--Moral and ethical aspects.
 4. Harm reduction. 5. Feminism and science.
 I. Title II. Seear, Kate.
 362.1'963623-dc22

Library of Congress Cataloging-in-Publication Data
Fraser, Suzanne, 1967-
 Making disease, making citizens : the politics of hepatitis C / by Suzanne
Fraser and Kate Seear.
   p. cm.
 Includes index.
 ISBN 978-1-4094-0839-0 (hardback)
 1. Hepatitis C--Social aspects. 2. Hepatitis C--Political
aspects. I. Seear, Kate. II. Title.

 RC848.H425F73 2011
 362.196'3623--dc23

                                                            2011027182
 ISBN 978-1-4094-0839-0 (hbk)
 ISBN 978-1-138-26834-0 (pbk)

Contents

List of Figures

Acknowledgements

This book is based on a research project funded by the Australian Research Council. The authors were based in the School of Political and Social Inquiry in the Faculty of Arts at Monash University, Melbourne, Australia. Suzanne Fraser's research and writing was also undertaken during a period spent at the National Centre in HIV Social Research at the University of New South Wales, Australia. Suzanne is a visiting fellow at the NCHSR and gratefully acknowledges the hospitality and support she received during the six months she spent there.

The chief investigators on the project from which the book emerges were Suzanne Fraser, Carla Treloar (based at the NCHSR) and David Moore (based at the National Drug Research Institute, Curtin University, Perth, Australia). We thank Carla and David for their contributions to the research project as a whole and for their valuable professional insights into drug use and hepatitis C.

Importantly, the study was anchored in 30 in-depth interviews with people diagnosed with hepatitis C. We are extremely grateful to our interview participants for their generosity in agreeing to talk to us about their experiences. Recruiting these participants and conducting the interviews was a major task requiring detailed knowledge of the area, tact and perseverance, and we are indebted to Emily Lenton for undertaking this key part of the research. We are also indebted to Hepatitis Victoria for their invaluable assistance with recruitment. Emily also coordinated the collection of health promotion literature, medical journal articles and self-help books and, overall, made an invaluable contribution to the study through her impressive knowledge of the area and her unerring sensitivity and insight into the lives and experiences of people with hepatitis C.

Of course, each of us also drew support and inspiration from different friends and colleagues. *Accordingly, Suzanne would like to express her gratitude to the following people.*

My first debt of gratitude is owed to Kate Seear, whose skill, humour and energy made writing this book a pleasure. Kate is an exceptionally talented scholar able to bring to her work a rare mix of analytical acuity, creativity and pragmatism. She is also a great friend who has been very much missed since her move to the United Kingdom during the final stages of writing this book. For much appreciated companionship and advice at the NCHSR, I thank Carla Treloar, Max Hopwood, Asha Persson, Jeanne Ellard, Dean Murphy, Jake Rance and Joanne Bryant. I am also very grateful for the friendship and support offered by the following people: Robyn Dwyer, Celia Roberts, kylie valentine, Gina Thomson, Rebecca Winter, Mark Davis, Narelle Miragliotta, Steven Angelides, JaneMaree Maher and Jo Lindsay. For so many acts of kindness, care and generosity, I thank David Moore. Louise Fraser, Jason Fraser, Michelle Fraser, Jane Caldwell and John Jacobs have given all the best things family can, and more.

Kate would also like to add the following acknowledgements.

First and most of all, I would like to thank Suzanne, who invited me to join her in this project. No words can describe how much I have gained from the opportunity to work with someone so genuinely passionate about academic work in general and hepatitis C in particular. Throughout this process, Suzanne has remained open to ideas, she has an extraordinary work ethic, an endless enthusiasm and a deep commitment to the capacity of academic work to make a difference. I could think of no better person to have worked with. She has been an absolute inspiration throughout this research and has become a very dear friend. I would also like to thank a number of people who contributed in some way to the research. The preparation of this book benefitted from my location within a community of like-minded researchers. To this end I give special thanks to Robyn Dwyer, Emily Lenton, David Moore, Carla Treloar and Rebecca Winter, all of whom I met in the course of this research. As well as their valuable intellectual contributions and constant encouragement, I have come to regard each of them as a great friend. I am, as you all know, mad keen. Thanks also go to colleagues from across Australia and the United Kingdom who were involved at various stages in discussions about the book, providing valuable feedback and encouragement, raising helpful suggestions or introducing challenging questions which have undoubtedly strengthened the analysis. These include Pete Higgs, Paul Dietze, Celia Roberts, kylie valentine, Helen Keane, Max Hopwood, Steven Angelides and Mark Davis. I would also like to thank my friends and family, especially my good friends at Monash University, Marina Cominos, Ben Whiteley, Zareh Ghazarian, Nick Economou and Narelle Miragliotta, whose humour and friendship sustained me during the writing process. And finally, my biggest thanks go to my sister Claire Seear, who was tasked with the hardest job of all: living with me while this book was written. Claire has been extraordinarily patient and supportive during the challenging writing process, and for that I am forever grateful.

Parts of the chapters to follow have already appeared in print. We are grateful to acknowledge the publishers' permission to include them. Sections of Chapter 3 appeared in Fraser, S. 2010. More than one and less than many: Materialising hepatitis C and injecting drug use in self-help literature and beyond. *Health Sociology Review*, 19(2), 230-44. Sections of Chapter 4 appeared in Fraser, S. 2010. Hepatitis C and the limits of medicalisation and biological citizenship for people who inject drugs. *Addiction Research & Theory*, 18(5), 544-56. In addition, a section on theoretical approaches to studying disease that appears in the Introduction first appeared in Fraser, S. (2011). Beyond the 'potsherd': The role of injecting drug use-related stigma in shaping hepatitis C. In Fraser, S.

and Moore, D. (eds). *The Drug Effect: Health, Crime and Society*. Melbourne: Cambridge University Press. We are also grateful to Hepatitis Queensland for permission to use artwork by Rachel Otto from their publication 'Bloody Little Factbook'.

Collaborations take a range of forms, and ours involved a planning process followed by the largely independent authoring of chapters. This writing stage was then combined with discussion and further writing as we worked towards bringing the chapters together. Suzanne wrote the Introduction, Chapters 1, 3, 4 and the Conclusion, while Kate wrote Chapters 2 and 5.

Introduction

A Gathering

Hepatitis C is a relatively newly identified but heavily stigmatised disease. Closely linked with injecting drug use and symbolically associated with HIV, its naming in 1989 gave shape to experiences of illness for many, but in so doing instantly created an abjected, stigmatised population. Since then, the form, meaning and implications of hepatitis C have been subject to continual debate, both within medicine and beyond it. As Robert Aronowitz argues, 'new consensus about illness is usually reached as a result of negotiations among the different parties with a stake in the outcome' (1998: 1). He emphasises that this process of negotiation is primarily social. This book maps the social and medical negotiations taking place around hepatitis C, and sheds light on the ways these negotiations have also co-produced new selves for those affected by the disease. The book also illuminates a set of broader issues relating to disease: how it is constituted in practice, how the ways in which it is constituted shapes lives, how knowledge about it authorises new subjects and new relationships. As we will argue, within contemporary neo-liberal societies the making of disease is also necessarily the making of subjects, of rights and of responsibilities. In that disease can be made and remade multiply (Mol 2002) we also ask how this disease can be remade to create new spaces of subjectivity.

Hepatitis C is a major health problem around the world. In Australia, where the study from which this book emerges was based, 2007 saw approximately 11,760 new diagnoses, and an estimated 207,600 people (over 1 per cent of the population) are now infected with the disease (National Centre in HIV Epidemiology and Clinical Research 2008a). Hepatitis C affects an estimated 120 to 170 million people worldwide (the World Health Organisation estimate of prevalence puts the rate at 2 per cent, or about 123 million people) (Shepard et al. 2005). It is the leading cause of liver transplantation in developed countries, and the most common chronic blood-borne infection in the United States. Infection occurs as a result of blood-to-blood contact. Most new infections in the West – up to 91 per cent in Australia – occur among people who inject drugs (National Centre in HIV Epidemiology and Clinical Research 2005) but historically infection has also occurred via blood transfusion and other forms of blood-to-blood contact including accidents, needle-stick injury, sharing of toothbrushes and so on. The effects of the disease are diverse but can be serious. As with other forms of hepatitis, the virus affects the liver. It is documented as able to cause day-to-day problems such as pain, fatigue and depression, as well as long term problems such as cirrhosis of the liver and liver cancer.[1]

---

1   The Australian Government's Department of Health and Ageing web site lists the following prognoses for hepatitis C based on 'available evidence thus far'. Of 100 people

Preventing transmission and dealing with the long-term effects of hepatitis C are pressing concerns. As Jacalyn Duffin (2005: 83) has argued, from the point of view of medical knowledge, hepatitis C is still very much 'under construction'. By this she means that, isolated as recently as 1989, the hepatitis C virus still presents many uncertainties to scientists (for example, in relation to natural history, treatment outcomes, and rates of spontaneous 'clearing' [or cure]). Hepatitis C is also very much under construction culturally and politically. Its association with injecting drug use creates a powerful net of meanings that help shape understandings of the disease and of prevention and treatment options. Further, the illicit status of injecting drug use both reflects and contributes to stigmatisation, as well as contributing to the scale and shape of the epidemic. The connection often assumed between HIV and hepatitis C in hepatitis C prevention and among people who inject drugs also contributes to the ways in which the disease is seen and dealt with. Subtended, then, by two heavily stigmatised phenomena[2] – injecting drug use (IDU) and HIV – this relatively new disease is being constructed along intensely politicised lines. How might this process of construction be understood? Hepatitis C differs from HIV in countless ways, one of them being that its cultural, social and political constitution is yet to be analysed by scholars in the same depth. This is an urgent task given that the disease affects increasing numbers of people and is associated with damaging social as well as health effects. This book represents an initial contribution to this task. It explores the construction of hepatitis C by drawing on a range of sources including 30 in-depth interviews conducted with people with hepatitis C; medical texts providing accounts of the development of knowledge about hepatitis C; hepatitis C prevention education literature (both current and early), and self-help books on hepatitis C (for example, *Living with Hepatitis C for Dummies* 2005). In doing so, the book plays two main roles. First, it offers the first social science book-length work on this symbolically and materially potent epidemic. Second, it performs a political analysis of disease. In this capacity the analysis offers insights we regard as at least partly translatable into a range of

---

with hepatitis C: about 65 to 85 people will develop chronic hepatitis C infection; about 5 to 10 of these will have progressed to cirrhosis after 20 years; about 3 to 5 of these risk liver failure or hepatocellular carcinoma after 30 to 40 years; the majority of people with chronic infection will probably not progress to advanced liver disease but their quality of life may be diminished. Associated with chronic infection are long-term symptoms such as fatigue, impaired cognitive function, low-grade fever, appetite and digestive problems, myalgia, depression and anxiety (St John and Sandt 2005, Hopwood and Treloar 2005). Thus, hepatitis C as it is currently understood entails relatively low rates of fatality and relatively high rates of chronic illness.

2   Throughout this book the terms 'phenomenon' and 'phenomena' will be used generally to refer to objects, emotions, ideas, practices and so on. These terms are taken from the work of Karen Barad, whose innovative feminist approach to materiality, which she describes as 'agential-realism', has been elaborated in detail elsewhere (2008) by Suzanne Fraser This terminology is used here because its epistemological and ontological implications closely articulate with the theoretical approach of the book.

other health contexts, and relevant to the study of other illnesses, health issues and health movements. In fulfilling this dual purpose the book draws on contemporary social theory, including Nikolas Rose's concept of biological citizenship, and John Law and Annemarie Mol's formulation of complexity.

In his 2007 book *The Politics of Life Itself* (2007) Nikolas Rose argues that health and illness are no longer simply polarised. Instead, individuals have become part of a mode of subjectification in which the continual pursuit of self improvement is expected. In this context, it is no longer acceptable to say, 'I am not ill, therefore I am well, and this is enough'. According to Rose, contemporary society encourages us to see ourselves as always open to somatic improvement, as well as to its opposite: ill health and physical decline. This perspective, along with the technologies developed in reflecting and promulgating it, open new avenues of both hope and fear in our lives. As Rose argues, the expectation that we must continually act to safeguard and enhance our health and our somatic integrity, combined with the expectation that we will do so voluntarily and as an expression of our 'true' selves, is an important way in which what he calls biological citizenship is constituted. This book draws on Rose's account of the developing relations between biomedicine and contemporary selves, considering it from the unique location occupied by hepatitis C-positive injecting drug users. How do injunctions to care for the self impact on these individuals? How well do Rose's observations about the rewards of biological citizenship fit this group? The analysis we conduct in this book both makes use of, and attempts to move beyond, Rose's approach.

The book also draws on the innovative approaches to method offered in the work of John Law, and in his collaborations with Annemarie Mol. Law's book, *After Method: Mess in Social Science Research* (2004) offers a range of insights into social science research useful for the analysis conducted for this book. Emerging from the generative encounter between feminist science studies and science and technology studies, Law's work takes as its aim the development of a new vocabulary for method, one that embraces rather than ignores or suppresses the elusive, the disorderly and the chaotic in research. In its ability to address some of the complexities inherent both in the method proposed for this book (its mixing of oral and textual sources, its desire to combine analysis of local, individual experiences and global debates about the nature of disease and the impact of medicalisation) and in the particular character of hepatitis C and what is currently known about it, this vocabulary will partly shape this book. As we will explain below, his collaboration with Mol on the edited collection *Complexities* (2002) also informs the book's approach and analysis.

Hepatitis C in the social sciences

To date, no book-length works analysing hepatitis C from a cultural or social perspective have been published. This contrasts starkly with the HIV research field, which is richly populated with sophisticated social and cultural analyses of the disease and of its impact on society and those affected by it (see for example Altman 1986, Dowsett 1996, Ariss 1997, Treichler 1999). These works have been read widely, and have actively informed scholarly and policy understandings of key issues in the response to HIV such as sexuality, medicalisation, treatment regimes, and gay culture and sociality. With rates of hepatitis C transmission still comparatively high, stigma and discrimination widespread, and increasing numbers of affected individuals facing long-term symptoms and debilitating treatment side effects, there is a pressing need for book-length works that increase our understanding of the social and political forces shaping this disease, along with work that can help produce effective responses to it.

The stigma associated with injecting drug use and – by extension – hepatitis C is well established in the literature (Krug 1997, Fraser and Treloar 2006, Anti-Discrimination Board of NSW 2006, Harris 2005, Pugh 2008). This stigma can be found operating within policy, the media, and in particular, within health service delivery (Anti-Discrimination Board of NSW 2006). Analysing stigmatising responses to injecting drug use and hepatitis C in a key site for meaning-making around disease, the media, Pugh notes (2008: 386):

> [its] classification of people with hepatitis C as 'innocent victims' or as guilty perpetrators perpetuates beliefs about injecting drug use as inherently bad and detrimental to the health of individuals and the community in general. Even seemingly straightforward news stories exclude injecting drug users in subtle ways and contribute to the maintenance of social inequalities between different groups of people.

This awareness of the stigmatised nature of hepatitis C characterises much of the critical literature exploring the disease and its implications for people who inject drugs (for reviews of the analysis of stigma in social science explorations of hepatitis C, see Butt 2008 and Patterson et al. 2007).

Alongside these observations about stigma, the social sciences literature on hepatitis C offers insights into experiences of diagnosis, treatment and living with the disease (for a review of available literature, see Treloar and Rhodes 2009). Much attention is also paid to analyses which aim to uncover more effective ways of preventing disease transmission. In keeping with the observations Rose has made about the individualisation of health, many of these studies take as their uninterrogated starting point the idea that individuals can and must control their health and that reducing incidence is primarily an individual responsibility (see Fraser 2004, for a critique of this tendency, and Moore and Fraser 2006 for a consideration of the alternatives). Without wishing to deny the capacity for agency among those most directly affected by this disease in the West – people who inject drugs – this book explicitly resists this approach, preferring to map meaning, process and effects much more broadly, and to understand the forces shaping disease more broadly too. Disease deserves to be understood as complex, emergent and distributed. Indeed, effective and equitable responses depend upon such understandings. Moving beyond the sometimes oversimplifying accounts of this disease and its prevention requires, however, some significant shifts in perspective. Given the forceful production of active, responsible health subjectivity within contemporary Western healthcare, developing and sustaining such a shift requires conscious effort and new conceptual tools. These tools help us to recognise and give due weight to aspects of disease otherwise downplayed or ignored in conventional accounts.

Risking theory in an epidemic

As we have already noted, hepatitis C is found all over the world. This does not mean its distribution is even or consistent. Notwithstanding some important variations, it is possible to identify a pattern in hepatitis C infection. It clusters among the most impoverished, disadvantaged and stigmatised members of almost any population, be this a national population in which injecting drug use is vilified, or a global population in which some nations are under-resourced compared to others. This clustering can be understood in a range of ways. The choices that can be made between these ways go to the core theoretical concerns of this book. One of the key aims of the book is to formulate an approach to disease able to acknowledge the ways in which social and political forces – namely poverty, disadvantage and stigma – directly shape the disease hepatitis C. Our approach will not, however, take the form of the fairly commonplace argument that impoverished and disadvantaged people transmit and contract disease more freely than the privileged. This approach would suggest (at least) two assumptions:

1. Hepatitis C pre-exists the populations in which it manifests;
2. Such populations should be enjoined to change their ways to reduce the freedom with which this pre-existing disease of hepatitis C moves between and across bodies.

These ideas are insufficiently sophisticated to capture the interrelationship of bodies and viruses and the social in the making of disease. They can also lead to insufficiently careful and effective strategies for responding to particular formulations of the problem of disease.

In an attempt to overcome the limitations of these assumptions, the book mobilises a set of theoretical concepts emerging from the work of science and technology studies and feminist studies scholars. Together (and to paraphrase), these critics argue that, contrary to conventional wisdom, diseases are not self-evident objects lying around waiting to be discovered. Instead they are emergent phenomena, constantly being made and remade by social forces. As we will demonstrate throughout the book, this approach to disease allows us to scrutinise legal, policy and social responses to hepatitis C in terms that identify the role of these phenomena in *making hepatitis C as disease*, and in *making people with the disease as certain types of citizens and non-citizens.* In short, the approach to disease proposed here denaturalises it, undermining the common view of it as essentially given in nature and, in that sense, possessed of intrinsic material attributes that determine its shape, actions and effects. In so doing it also disrupts the notion that a disease's subjects pre-exist the disease and that those subjects determine the disease's shape, actions and effects.

According to Jacalyn Duffin (2005: 32), diseases do not just *impact on* society and culture. They are also partially constituted by society and culture. Speaking explicitly about hepatitis C, she asserts that:

> Diseases are not immutable objects lying around waiting to be unearthed like potsherds in an archaeological dig. The so-called discoverer of a disease has actually 'elaborated', 'recognised', 'described' or 'invented' a new way of understanding a problem that has previously been overlooked or forgotten, possibly because it had not been considered a problem.

In Duffin's view, disease concepts theorise illness; its origins, location and the nature of its activity. Duffin notes, for example, that Western medicine is dominated by the organismic concept of disease, which understands disease as a discontinuous state located in the individual. It seems, then, hepatitis C can be seen not as a corporeal 'potsherd' simply dug up and described by medical researchers, but a socially constituted object our responses to which materially shape it over time. What are the implications of this? Most pressingly, seeing disease this way invites the recognition that political forces and events are part of this process of materialisation. If this is the case, engaging with these political forces and events becomes a necessary way in which to try to reshape disease and ameliorate its effects.

In taking up the question of the sufficiency of current theoretical approaches to disease and the need for greater sophistication in our concepts, we could well attract criticism for directing our focus away from the all-important, sometimes heartbreaking, material conditions of disease, and lived experiences of these epidemics. This would, of course, be far from our intention. Our aim here is to demonstrate the direct links between concepts and materiality and to make an explicit contribution to practices which bear immediately on the lives of those affected by hepatitis C. This is not, of course, an easy task. Paula Treichler has attended closely to the issue in her highly influential 1999 book, *How to Have Theory in an Epidemic: Cultural Chronicles of AIDS.* Treichler opens her book by asking, 'What should be the role of theory in an epidemic?' (1999: 3). She goes on to note that (1999: 3):

> The very mention of theory, cultural construction or discourse may be exasperating or distressing to those face to face with the epidemic's enormity and overwhelming practical demands.

Treichler's focus is HIV, not hepatitis C, and it is important to recall that her comments are made in relation to a life-threatening disease that goes untreated among the vast majority of those affected around the world. Mortality rates for HIV are extremely high in parts of Africa and elsewhere and those who contract the disease can face very short futures when unable to access treatment. It would not do to conflate the circumstances of HIV with those of hepatitis C. This is not, however, to say that hepatitis C is not a serious disease warranting serious attention and resourcing. As we have noted, it can significantly limit quality of life and lead to severe liver disease, and treatment options are at present quite limited. While those able to access treatment for HIV cannot hope for cure, they can look forward to long lives with disease progression and symptoms very effectively managed. By contrast, those able to access hepatitis C treatment – a combination of the drugs interferon and ribavirin – face the possibility of cure, but if this is not achieved through treatment (itself extremely onerous and debilitating) no medical treatment is available to manage symptoms and disease progression. Clearly the two diseases diverge markedly in their relationships to medicine, but both are serious health conditions and major public health issues. It is in this sense that Treichler's work on epidemics informs the argument made here, especially given that HIV and hepatitis C are both diseases profoundly characterised by stigma and discrimination.

Just as Treichler unequivocally argues for the importance of theory in the face of HIV-related disaster, we argue for the importance of theory for engaging effectively with the scale and seriousness of hepatitis C incidence and prevalence. As Treichler asserts in countering the tendency to polarise 'theory' and 'real life' (1999: 3): 'theory *is* about "people's lives"' (emphasis added). As she points out, we need to examine the representation of disease because representation is never less than part of the process of constitution (1999: 4):

> Language is not a substitute for reality; it is one of the most significant ways we know reality, experience it, and articulate it.

Treichler's book tells an important story of the discursive (and thus, in turn, material) constitution of HIV. Chapter 1, for example, traces the early epidemiological decisions that constituted HIV as a 'gay' disease even as transmission via injecting drug use remained common. Treichler notes that HIV scholars and advocates held the view that the constitution of the disease as 'gay' delayed public health and other responses in the United States. This is an interesting point to consider in light of what is known about responses to hepatitis C. While there is little doubt the promulgation of the notion of the 'gay plague' affected public perceptions by shaping HIV as intrinsically immoral – and simultaneously as largely sequestered within a marginal population – it is unlikely that clarifying its connection with injecting drug use would have altered this perception. In that people who inject drugs were just as stigmatised and marginalised as gay men at the time, greater recognition of their vulnerability to or place in the epidemic would not necessarily have generated faster, more committed, or more effective responses. Still, there can be little argument that the construction of HIV as a gay disease shaped responses, and still plays a part in the West's inability to fully engage with the worldwide (overwhelmingly heterosexual) epidemic and its implications. In these ways, Treichler's work reminds us of the importance of theory, concepts and language in the material enactment of disease. Her analysis begins from the now well-recognised view that material objects such as disease should be seen as constructed, rather than as ontologically stable or foundational, and their attributes as contingent upon rather than anterior to social relations. In this respect Treichler's work draws on science and technology studies (STS). Indeed, it incorporates the early STS work of Bruno Latour and Steve Woolgar on the role of language and ideas in materialising objects: 'Interpretations do not so much *inform* as *perform*' (Latour and Woolgar quoted in Treichler 1999: 26, emphasis in the original).

In that Treichler's understanding of disease brackets the 'facts' of HIV as dependent upon the circumstances of the disease's constitution, it also raises questions about the status of facts themselves and the role of research in making facts. These issues are of central importance to this book. Our argument concerns the making of facts about hepatitis C, so it would not do to simply posit alternative facts about the disease. If we do not speak of facts and their replacement, however, what should we speak of? Here Latour (2004) assists us by proposing a shift in focus from 'matters of fact' to 'matters of concern'. Writing in the aftermath of the attack on the World Trade Center, Latour laments what he sees as the unfortunate similarity between some forms of critique of science and its facts and those conspiracy theories sometimes used to explain or dismiss world events such as the attack in question. He mentions global warming and our need to mobilise to arrest it, arguing that without facts we are not able to act in urgently required ways. He questions the direction of critique, and, in clarifying his own intentions in the work he has conducted to date, explains that he 'intended to emancipate the public from prematurely naturalised objectified facts' rather than to dismiss facts altogether as unnecessary or utterly without validity. Interestingly, given the subject of this book, he figures the role of the critic in the following terms (2004: 231):

> ...we behaved like mad scientists who have let the virus of critique out of the confines of their laboratories and cannot do anything now to limit its deleterious effects; it mutates now, gnawing everything up, even the vessels in which it is contained.

Here critique is a 'virus': an uncontrollable destructive force if not properly contained. It is an intrinsically dangerous phenomenon that if used as a tool, can generate knowledge, but can easily exceed this brief and become simply destructive. Against this destructiveness, Latour asserts that (2004: 231), 'The question was never to get away from facts but closer to them, not fighting empiricism but on the contrary, renewing empiricism'. He wants in turn to salvage realism, but to remake it in doing so. He argues, therefore, for a shift from a preoccupation with 'matters of fact' to one with 'matters of concern'. What is the difference? 'Matters of fact are only very partial ... and very polemical, very political, renderings of matters of concern' (2004: 232). Facts, he asserts, are made by social and political processes and can only ever describe issues, objects and events in very partial and shallow ways. The role of the critic, he says, is to develop new ways of addressing matters of concern rather than mobilising and creating more matters of fact. In doing so, critics should aim not to 'debunk' but, following Donna Haraway, to 'protect and care'.

These observations usefully address the issue this book tackles – how, that is, to frame disease more effectively so as to better understand and address the role of politics in its making. Hepatitis C can, we argue, be seen as a 'matter of concern' instead of a matter of fact. Speaking of the facts of hepatitis C in their pre-critical sense as though the facts as they are currently constituted, selected and communicated are all there is, will not do. Nor, however, will simply disposing of facts as though the disease, its implications and those affected by it have no material existence. Instead, following Latour, we might think of hepatitis C as a 'thing' in the Heideggerian sense – a gathering that exceeds any notion of simple fact or object. The word 'thing', Latour points out, has its origins in old Icelandic, which also uses it to refer to forms of Parliament – to what he describes as (2004: 233) 'the oldest of the sites in which our ancestors did their dealing and tried to settle their disputes'. The thing, then, is both 'an object out there' and 'an issue very much in here, at any rate, a gathering'. Things, in this sense, are as much made, or 'gathered', in culture and action as they are given prior to culture and action. If we are in any doubt as to the utility of this formulation of the difference between fact and concern, Latour asserts that 'Things that gather cannot be thrown at you like objects' (2004: 237). Anyone who knows anything about the social and political status of injecting drug use, and the stigma associated with hepatitis C, will surely recognise the strategic merits of this kind of approach. At present, for example, hepatitis C is mainly seen in the West as the 'result' of injecting drug use. As Harris (2005) has noted, the two are 'virtually conflated' in the scholarly literature, and in public health. Of course, there is a strong association between injecting and infection. In a microbial sense this association can to some degree be seen as causal. Yet, as the case of Egypt shows, the conflation of disease with injecting drug use is entirely circumstantial (See Fraser [2011] for a detailed discussion of this case). Egypt has an extremely high rate of infection as a result of nationally funded health campaigns that relied on non-sterile injecting practices (Frank et al. 2000). It is a hepatitis C epidemic no way confined to any kind of stigmatised activity. From this point of view, hepatitis C can be seen as a matter of concern, or a 'thing' in the Heideggerian sense – both material object and site of dealing and dispute, the facts entailed in which are constituted but no less real for this. In one place hepatitis C is synonymous with injecting illicit drugs, and with a series of social ills assumed to go along with injecting drug use, in another with well-intentioned public health initiatives aimed at protecting the population from disease. Following from this understanding of disease are at least two observations:

first, that the facts of disease can be understood as socially produced, and second, that they can be reproduced differently. Reproducing the facts of hepatitis C is important for a number of reasons:

1. The perceived causal relationship between the stigmatised practice of injecting drug use and the harms associated with hepatitis C may be loosened, reducing the scope for blaming those who contract the disease;
2. In turn this reduction in blame may allow responses more inclined to generosity and to broadly conceived networks of responsibility and action;
3. Where responses change, so does the disease itself. As has been argued already, diseases do not precede human action – they are made and remade within it.

In relation to this last point, Rosenberg (2002: 237) points out that the modern approach to illness sees diseases as 'entities existing outside the unique manifestations of illness in particular men and women'. A related observation can be made by replacing 'men and women' with 'social and cultural contexts'. The essentialising of disease, argues Rosenberg (2002: 238), allows medicine to enact, intentionally and incidentally, a range of normalising functions:

> Everywhere we see specific disease concepts being used to manage deviance, rationalise health policies, plan health care and structure specialty relationships within the medical profession.

Disease concepts of hepatitis C do precisely this, particularly as they essentialise causal factors and the character of affected populations at the same time as they essentialise disease itself. What have been the effects of the particular ways in which hepatitis C has been conceptualised in the West? One answer can be found in tracing the role of stigma in shaping hepatitis C. As Simmonds and Coomber (2009) argue in their analysis of stigma related to injecting drug use:

> In the public policy and health sphere the stigmatisation of specific populations may also result in the view that certain populations are less 'worthy' and therefore 'less eligible' or less 'deserving' of services than other groups.

While Simmonds' and Coomber's observations about stigma are highly relevant here, their approach to the problem and to its solutions tends to reproduce the approach this book aims to question. In considering how best to deal with stigma, they argue:

> The effects of stigma on IDU populations are sufficiently far-reaching for health care providers and others whose remit it is to reduce the harms emanating from injecting drug use, to seriously consider its impact, its production and how best to address the problems it causes.

If we proceed analytically in terms of 'matters of concern', we must see the facts associated with them as constituted socially, and their materiality as emergent rather than foundational. In this context we cannot position 'IDU populations' as anterior to stigma, and the 'effects' of stigma as separate from 'health care providers and others'. A 'matter of concern' approach treats the facts of the matter as emergent and contingent, and objects as 'things' – as always already sites of dealing and dispute. So the category 'IDU' and its characteristics do not meaningfully precede the operations of stigma, and the effects of stigma do not meaningfully precede the practices of health care providers and others. Injecting drug use, health care provision and stigma emerge continually in relation to each other, and hepatitis C too is produced through these phenomena, just as it contributes in turn to their production.

To bring the issues canvassed here together for broader purposes, our key point is that disease should not be taken for granted. It does not, as medicine tends to imply, lie in bodies passively awaiting discovery, description and mastery. Indeed, as in the case of Egypt, it is at times actively *made by medicine* and related agencies. This reframing of disease has important implications for our understanding of health, marginalisation and drug use. Where disease is not fully recognised as a 'thing': as always already both an object and a site of dealing and dispute, the importance and complex role of politics in actually making disease and those who have it cannot be fully recognised. So long, as Paula Treichler has argued, as reality and theory are seen as separate, and reality is seen to occupy its own autonomous form of existence anterior to theory, we will proceed as though disease is largely a pre-determined matter, the character and implications of which can only be addressed posterior to its manifestation. Our point, ultimately, is that conventions and values and social practices such as health policy and stigma make the disease as much as microbes do. Disease is a gathering, a matter of concern that far exceeds the 'facts' by which it can be described. It is made in many moments and in many ways, and as such is the responsibility – and the 'fault' – of many individuals, groups and forces, not just of those who 'have' it. When we consider how to view treatment, and how to provide it, these ideas are indispensable. Things that gather cannot be thrown at you like objects.

How can account based on the notion of gathering, an account that addresses the complexities of hepatitis C, best be written? Here, the work of Annemarie Mol and John Law is helpful (Law 1999, Mol 1999, Mol and Law 2002, Mol 2002, Law 2004). Drawing on a rich background in science and technology studies and feminist science studies, including of course the work of Latour, these theorists work in an area they sometimes refer to as 'ontics' or 'ontological politics'. In brief, these terms relate to an approach to knowledge and materiality that relates to constructionism but takes an extra crucial step beyond some of its key features. Constructionism contends that phenomena, including material objects and the 'natural world', are constituted by discourse and do not pre-exist society and culture (Goode and Ben-Yehuda 1994). This approach to reality has been embraced by scholars and others desiring to effect political transformation. If reality, even the natural world and material objects otherwise seen as immutable and given, is the product of discourse and the operations of social and cultural forces, it is amenable to change and cannot be used to justify existing social or political relations, existing social or political inequities and injustices. Annemarie Mol draws on this approach in her work on diseases, but in the course of her ethnographic research generates a new ontological claim beyond constructionist accounts. While constructionism recognises the 'made-ness' of apparently given things such as diseases, it tends to frame the processes of making as singular and terminal. That is, these processes happen once, come to an end and, as a result, we are left with a disease or other object constituted in a certain way: a product of its social and temporal context to be sure, but complete and now immutable in its constructedness. As Mol (1999: 76) points out:

> Constructivist stories suggest that alternative 'constructions of reality' might have been possible. They have been possible in the past, but vanished before they ever fully blossomed.

Against this view, Mol argues that, on the contrary, phenomena are always being made and remade – multiple processes of constitution occur at any given time, shaped and informed by the various discourses in which they are inserted (or from which they emerge). Mol traces these processes in her research into diabetes, atherosclerosis and anaemia. In relation to anaemia, she argues (1999: 79):

> The reality of anaemia takes various forms. These are not perspectives seen by different people … neither are they alternative, bygone constructions of which only one has emerged from the past … they are different versions, different performances, different realities that co-exist in the present.

For Mol, this claim that realities are constantly in the making, and that the moment of construction is never complete or behind us, underwrites the political purchase of her approach. She argues that from the point of view of ontological politics, four questions emerge about the constitution of realities:

1. Where are the options?
2. What is at stake?
3. Are there really options?
4. How should we choose?

Implicit in these questions is the assumption, rather like that addressed in Latour's work, that realities are always open to making and remaking – that is, reality is made of matters of concern. Such questions are intensely productive in the context of hepatitis C. With knowledge about genotypes, transmission, chronicity and treatment still highly volatile and unsettled, the options for those facing a diagnosis are by no means clear. With rates of success for treatment constantly under revision and knowledge about the long term effects of chronicity still in development as research continues past the first 20-year mark of disease naming, the stakes involved in diagnosis are by no means settled. With knowledge still seen as highly provisional, there is no doubt that many possibilities about how to proceed exist. Right now, in public meetings, professional gatherings and the media, those affected are engaged in processes of debate over how to choose between these options. No doubt, many of these options will be pursued simultaneously. In short, as with other apparently ahistorical, apolitical material phenomena, hepatitis C is not a fixed and given object with intrinsic material – and therefore political – attributes and implications. Neither is it a constituted object now possessing stable meanings and attributes. It is always already enacted: made in practice, or to take a term from the theories of performativity (Butler 1990, 1993) also inspiring Mol and Law (Law 1999, Mol 2002a), its ontology is iteration.

If this is the case, how then might disease be thought further? Here, Duffin's (2005) work offers valuable insights. According to Duffin, diseases should not be seen only to *impact on* society and culture. They are also partially *constituted by* society and culture. As we have already noted, Duffin rejects the idea of disease as 'potsherd', preferring to acknowledge the ways in which it constitutes an elaboration, description or invention of a new way of understanding a problem. Disease concepts theorise illness; its origins, location and the nature of its activity. In the process of theorising illness, disease concepts necessarily theorise affected individuals. If, then, hepatitis C can be seen not as a corporeal 'potsherd' simply dug up and described by medical researchers, but a continually iterated thing – the description, metaphorical representation and treatment of which materially shapes it over time and changes it over time – we are left with a very complex task in articulating it.[3] Each of our chapters aims to demonstrate this process and its effects, sometimes explicitly, sometimes implicitly, drawing on this theory to do so.

Hepatitis C: A gathering

Complex phenomena materialise in different ways, at different times, and in relation to many different forces, objects and ideas. The shape of this book, the

---

3   As the first author (Suzanne Fraser) has noted elsewhere (Fraser 2003), the notion of articulation is theorised in many ways (Deleuze and Guattari 1987, Donna Haraway 1992 and Stuart Hall 1996). In this book we rely on Haraway's formulation. She expresses a preference for the notion of articulation over that of representation, explaining that: 'Human beings use names to point to themselves and other actors and easily mistake the names for the things. These same humans also think the traces of inscription devices are like names-pointers to things, such that the inscriptions and the things can be enrolled in dramas of substitution and inversion. But the things, in my view, do not pre-exist as ever-elusive, but fully pre-packaged, referents for the names. Other actors are more like tricksters than that. Boundaries take provisional, never finished shape in articulatory practices' (1992: 313).

14   *Making Disease, Making Citizens*

order in which ideas emerge in it, reflects this complexity in several ways. First, the book makes no attempt to 'begin at the beginning' or to commence from a point understood to be the origin of the ideas and issues we trace and analyse. To understand the process in this way would risk reinstating a singular 'real' object of study – disease – the origin and trajectory of which can be neatly established and traced. Second, the book recognises that core issues such as stigma, the materialisation of disease, the responsibilised health subject and so on circulate across the domains in which our object emerges in many, often untidy, ways. For this reason, these key issues arise in the chapters in a range of modes, appearing and re-appearing, sometimes circling back on themselves in cycles of iteration, linking to other issues and concepts in new ways each time. Our aim is to build understanding across chapters but to do so in keeping with the idea of the 'walk' Mol and Law (2002) introduce so intriguingly. The walk is one of three modes Mol and Law recommend in analysing phenomena in ways that avoid the simplistic overview. The three are: lists, cases and walks. The aim of all three is to produce 'modes of relating that allow the simple to coexist with the complex, of aligning elements without necessarily turning them into a comprehensive system or a complete overview' (2002: 16). Lists, cases and walks produce accounts of the world as open and unordered, accounts that allow new possibilities to emerge. Of course, lists can sometimes operate as overviews where they 'impose a single mode of ordering' (2002: 14). The kind of list Mol and Law recommend is one for which no claim is made to comprehensiveness and in which the items are not presented hierarchically. Lists, if conceived appropriately, allow the loose arrangement of phenomena of different kinds and scales, placed together to open up thought about the relationships between each. Importantly, lists of this kind do not, in their structure, create closure. A new item can always be added at the bottom. Change, that is, can be accommodated and even anticipated.

Cases are objects of analysis that have epistemological utility without laying claim to representativeness. In this book we treat hepatitis C as a 'case'. As Mol and Law (2002) explain, cases allow the following:

1. They sensitise us to otherwise unrecognised events and situations;
2. Offer potentially 'translatable' ideas and insights;
3. In disrupting assumptions they can 'destabilise expectations';
4. They can be used as allegory, to speak indirectly about other things.

In short, cases are both sensitising and unique. This book aims to use hepatitis C as a case in all these ways. Our exploration is first and foremost directed at better thinking through this particular disease in its complexity, the issues and questions and challenges associated with it, but it is also about treating hepatitis C as a case for disease (and for phenomena more broadly) where appropriate. And walks? Inspired by the work of Michel de Certeau, Mol and Law (2002) explain that the 'walk' is a means of moving through a space without relying upon or generating an overview. Phenomena are encountered within the space in a spontaneous and not necessarily orderly way. These can be drawn together, or left separate, depending upon the aim of the walk. To walk, and tell stories about, terrain, is their goal, rather than to make maps and produce seamless accounts of reality.

This book's intention is to walk and tells stories about hepatitis C. It would not be quite right to say that, based on Mol and Law's ideas, we have actively suppressed the development of an overview of the topic of the book. In writing, we have made meaning for ourselves and hopefully for others, and to a degree, the ordering of this meaning into an overview, is unavoidable. Of course, Mol and Law's point is not so much that overviews can be 'nipped in the bud' and never allowed to take hold. Rather, an overview, authoritative and comprehensive though it might seem, must always be recognised as necessarily partial and dependent on circumstance. It always creates 'presence, manifest absence and otherness' (Law 2004: 84). If an overview cannot ever be exhaustive or complete, if it cannot ever hope to finally, if built perfectly, capture reality correctly once and for all, it follows that no 'proper' structure exists for that overview. Certainly, a traditional linear structure that would work to erase the processes by which ideas and objects emerge in research and in our growing understanding, is one option. The option we have chosen to take is not the opposite of this, in that it does not seek to enact chaos. Yet it departs from it intentionally. Beginning in the middle, it follows the data, the issues and the ideas where they lead, and works to bring them together in meaning making without placing (what our theoretical approach leads us to judge) undue emphasis on traditional conceptual ordering narrative devices such as origins, causes, effects and so on. As Bruno Latour (2005) reminds us, collectivities are the effects, rather than the origins, of social processes. 'Society', to take his core example, does not make things happen as much as it is the effect of sometimes concerted, sometimes incidental, happenings. To use Law's term, society is 'gathered', that is, brought together through processes exceeding those taken for granted in normative epistemological models based on consistency and coherence (see Law 2004 for more). As with society, so too with hepatitis C, stigma, the citizen and so on. This 'walk' among the issues, processes and gatherings we have followed through our data and our animating concepts will, we hope, illuminate and prompt reflection without claiming to offer a comprehensive or complete account of the subject.

The book begins by following the development of concepts of hepatitis C in a specific sub-set of medical literature. In this first chapter we analyse those accounts that aim for precisely the perspective we question ourselves – that of the 'overview'. Since 1989 when 'hepatitis C' was first mobilised as a name for a set of viruses and a disease, articles summarising knowledge about the disease have appeared regularly in the medical literature, emerging from a range of medical specialties. Analysing these articles at the beginning of the book provides some valuable opportunities but also carries with it a risk of misunderstanding. In this chapter we begin our project in the middle of an important discursive domain for our object of study. Medicine is a key site of meaning making for hepatitis C. It is not, of course, the *origin* of meaning making for this disease, and we do not treat it as such. To suggest it were would be to understand medicine naively as neutral: as anterior to the social processes of meaning making. Instead we look at the ways in which stigma both animates and emerges from the material. To do this, we experimentally mobilise the medical terminology of hepatitis C 'quasispecies' to form a temporary set of analytic tools. Annemarie Mol and John Law's work on complexity (2002) forms the inspiration for this task. By refracting the notion of quasispecies through feminist theory, we build an approach that emphasises the productivity of error, multiplicity and contingency, exposing as we go the literature's desire to assert the opposite: scientific ideals of certainty, unity and autonomy.

The second chapter builds on this starting point by examining an area – hepatitis C-related health promotion – directly connected to the medical literature on hepatitis C in that it treats medicine as the key source of appropriate knowledge and content for its own aims. The health promotion literature we analyse can be examined for many different purposes. In our case, we have chosen to address it to a question equally relevant to each of the areas explored in this book: according to this discourse, what *is* hepatitis C? This is an important question for the book's purposes because as we will argue, hepatitis C as 'disease state' is constituted in action; its ontology is thoroughly political. The health promotion literature is a particularly valuable place to trace this process of constitution because it mobilises both the authority of science, and some of the techniques of popular media. Health promotion articulates (with) medical knowledge via images and textual strategies aimed at easy and effective public consumption. As it does so, it reshapes medical knowledge through its own imperatives, assumptions and unexamined figures and conventions. Its explicit intention is that readers adopt and act upon the injunctions it crafts from these articulations.[4] Prefiguring some of the arguments made later in the book about the role of hepatitis C in delineating and evoking certain forms of citizenship, the chapter concludes that health promotion demands 'excellence' in the form of enterprise, individuality, autonomy and responsible action.

Another discursive domain in which medical knowledge of hepatitis C is accorded a central place is that of self-help. While health promotion literature sometimes incorporates common features of the self-help genre, it differs from conventional self-help in that it is not commercially produced and is usually much less detailed, most often taking the form of leaflets and other short documents rather than books. Health promotion is produced by government and related bodies and is directly linked to public health imperatives, while self-help is most explicitly directed toward individual health and well-being. Chapter 3 looks closely at hepatitis C-related self-help books, highlighting these points of overlap and difference as it conducts its main line of enquiry – how hepatitis C and those who have the disease are materialised in this literature, and what effects these

---

4　Law (2005) defines 'crafting' as 'the enactment and condensation of presence in method assemblage'. Not necessarily limited to human agency, crafting occurs with all phenomena – nothing is given in nature, nothing is anterior to social relations.

materialisations have on individual daily lives and broader understandings of drug use, infectious disease and stigma. The chapter draws on Mol and Law's discussions of complexity in social science research to conduct its analysis, concluding that there are many ways in which responses to the disease, attempts to alleviate stigma and impact positively on individual health and well-being in this literature articulate key phenomena in the very ways that produce the problems of stigma and blame themselves. How best to intervene in these complex loops to interrupt their negative effects? This issue is also discussed via Mol and Law's provocative ideas about complexity.

Chapters 4 and 5 move from the analysis of textual sources to the interpretation of face-to-face interviews we conducted with people who have at one time or another been diagnosed with hepatitis C. Again we do not, of course, aim to reproduce a presumed pattern of causation in the order of this book's chapters – to assume that textual discourse emerges prior to the constitution of individual subjects and thus shapes their speech such that examining them first makes most sense. We do, however, consider our analysis of broader medical, health promotion and self-help literatures as useful in sketching out key threads of meaning through and with which our interview participants must weave their understandings of disease and constitute selves in relation to disease. These two final chapters will, therefore, draw on the themes identified in earlier chapters in developing specific arguments about individual experiences of hepatitis C.

In the first of these final chapters, we discuss the pivotal medical and social moment of diagnosis. We look at the particular dynamics that operate when people who inject drugs are diagnosed with hepatitis C and simultaneously become the targets of contemporary injunctions to preventive health and self-care. We note first that these medicalised subjects attract competing characterisations: their status as 'addicts' sees them medicalised as illegitimate risk takers suffering from a 'disease of the will' and thus lacking self-control, while their status as hepatitis C patients medicalises them in quite a different way: as potentially responsible self-regulating health consumers necessarily open to taking legitimate corporeal risks, such as those courted in treatment. We go on to address a pressing question that emerges directly from this tension: how do people who inject drugs respond to the contrary and intensely morally inflected injunctions to biological citizenship thrown up by the collision of two key ideological notions: addiction and infectious disease?

The second of the interview-based chapters, and the final chapter in the book, explores treatment for hepatitis C. Entailed in diagnosis is a process of enrolment into medical care, and, in turn, into a deliberative relationship with those 'solutions' to hepatitis C offered by medicine such as treatment. While Chapter 4 also raises treatment as a means of considering the claim to authority attendant upon medicalising responses to hepatitis C diagnosis, this chapter takes a more thorough look at the issue, focusing on how pathways into treatment perform subjects. In this, the chapter draws together observations made throughout the book about the political character of disease, the discursive constitution of medical optimism and the responsibility to act in relation to the opportunities presented in medical enactments of disease. The book's overall approach is built on the recognition that the constitution of subjectivity is thoroughly political, contingent, and emergent in action. Where subjectivity can be seen as co-constituted by disease, we must ask how the politics of disease – here of hepatitis C – and its contingencies and conditions of enactment shape subjectivity. Looking specifically at a key site of this process of co-constitution, treatment, we ask: if we take hepatitis C as a thoroughly political object, what do we make of efforts to treat the virus? How, in short, might we conceptualise the relationship between subject, treatment and politics?

Together the analyses conducted in each chapter build a series of sketches intended to expand our understanding of this disease and the processes and forces shaping it. Determined to live with complexity, we will not conclude the book with an overview or tidy set of recommendations, although we will certainly make statements aimed at contributing to change. Within these pages we have tracked the stigma associated with hepatitis C, prompted by past research in the field. We have also asked questions about the production of stigma, and explored the ways in which it is made and remade in responses to the disease – responses that are, at the same time, enactments of it. In this sense we do our best to attend to Latour's advice in his book *Reassembling the Social* (2005). In this work Latour takes sociologists to task for taking for granted the very object it is their job to explain. In our book hepatitis C, disease, stigma and so on all need to be explained even as we take them for granted as the starting points for our analysis. We hold both at once and in so doing hope to do all a simple text can in respecting complexity (Mol and Law 2002: 6).

Chapter 1
Towards a Quasispecies Epistemology

As we have already noted, medical discourse is an important mechanism through which meanings about hepatitis C are constituted and deployed in culture. In this chapter we begin our sketch of the disease by exploring medical articulations of hepatitis C in the form of review and summary articles tracking developments in knowledge about the virus. We track a key theme through the articles over time – that of scientific progress – noting how discussions of the knowability and containability of the disease, the framing of transmission and the action of testing have changed, and thinking through the meaning and effects of these changes. Our purpose is to offer a first sketch of an approach to knowledge – an epistemology – that helps bring to light some of the forces shaping understandings of the disease and of people who have it. Annemarie Mol and John Law's work on complexity (2002) forms the inspiration for the chapter's conceptual focus – one that takes the highly medicalised concept of virus 'quasispecies' and refracts it through feminist theory to provide a set of tools for understanding hepatitis C in its social and political complexity. As Mol and Law argue, it is all too easy to criticise 'oversimplification' when it comes to understanding social forces, and all too easy to observe that our objects of study are complex. All research, they say, needs to simplify in order to produce coherent accounts of things, but the key task is to stay alert to the complexities lost in these accounts, to build into our methods ways of keeping our eyes on both. This chapter is a starting point for work of this kind. It develops a way of thinking about knowledge production, and epistemology, built on both theoretical and material phenomena.

In generating the analysis presented in this chapter we looked at 29 articles chosen as general reviews, overviews and updates published across a range of medical specialties including hepatology, virology and immunology.[1] Between

---

1 These articles are: Bhandari, B.N. and Wright, T.L. (1995); Bonkovsky, H.L. and Mehta, S. (2001); Carey, W.D. and Patel, G. (1992); Colquhoun, S.D. (1996); Forns, X., Bukh, J. and Purcell, R.H. (2002); Fung, S.K. and Lok, A.S.F. (2005); Harvey, A.J. and Harvey, K.G. (2008); Hughes, C.A. and Shafran, S.D. (2006); Hwang, S-J. (2001); Gutfreund, K.S. and Bain, V.G. (2000); Lindsay, K.L. (1997); Maddrey, W.C. (2001); Moradpour, D., Cerny, A., Heim, M.H. and Blum, H.E. (2001); Pearlman, B.L. (2004a); Pearlman, B.L. (2004b); Plagemann, P. (1991); Purcell, R.H. (1997); Purcell, R.H. (2006); Sarbah, S.A. and Younossi, Z.M. (2000); Sarrazin, C. (2004); Sharara, A.I., Hunt, C.M. and Hamilton, J.D. (1996); Sherlock, S. (1996); Smith, B.C., Strasser, S.I. and Desmond, P.V. (1995); Walker, M.A. (1999); Walker, M.P., Appleby, T.C., Zhong, W., Lau, J.Y.N. and Hong, Z. (2003); Walsh, K. and Alexander, G.J.M. (2001); Woerz, I., Lohmann, V. and

November 2008 and March 2010, online searches of three databases (Medline, PubMed and Google Scholar) were conducted. The keywords used to conduct the searches were: 'review', 'overview', 'history', 'knowledge', 'progress', 'evolution', 'current perspectives', 'new', 'to date' and 'what we know'. Links to the 'related' articles and references lists from those articles identified were also followed. A total of 72 medical journal articles charting the history of the identification of hepatitis C and the growing knowledge about various aspects of hepatitis C were sourced. From this list, articles covering the main issues on hepatitis C research and development (nature of the virus, diagnosis, testing and treatment) with the words 'review' and 'overview' in the heading were selected for analysis, as well as the medical histories documenting the 'discovery' of the virus. This produced the corpus of 29 articles analysed for this chapter.

Towards a quasispecies epistemology

This chapter explores what we will call a 'quasispecies epistemology'. Its aim is to analyse key features of the construction of hepatitis C through a figurative mobilisation of the virology term 'quasispecies'. It does this as a means of enacting Mol and Law's proposal that complexity and simplification need to be held simultaneously if new, more productive analyses of social phenomena are to be produced. The chapter begins with a discussion of the notion of quasispecies, one which makes links with central aspects of Mol and Law's critique of complexity. In conducting this discussion, the chapter distinguishes a medical ontology of quasispecies from a critical feminist ontology. Despite the differences between the two ontologies that emerge in this discussion, it will be argued that the notion of quasispecies can illuminate how phenomena located at the intersection of stigma, (medical) epistemic uncertainty and political volatility, as is hepatitis C, function to shape marginalised lives and are in turn shaped by them.

What can a thoroughly medical concept such as that of 'quasispecies' offer a feminist critique of medicine? This depends on how the concept is handled and to what end it is engaged. As mobilised in medical accounts of hepatitis C, the notion of quasispecies operates mainly as a means of describing an aspect of what is taken, in the most realist of terms, to be an *a priori* material object. At the same time, however, it is a way of understanding viruses, individuals, groups and processes, and as such can be used in an ontological experiment, provoking a series of political observations about hepatitis C. What does it mean, for instance, to say as did the *Journal of Virology* in 1992 (Martell et al. 66:5), that hepatitis C circulates as a 'population', or as the *Journal of Molecular Biology* did much more recently (Más et al. 2010: 866), as a 'clan'? In the first place, we can see that this statement could be understood in the terms drawn from the work of Mol and

Bartenschlager, R. (2009); Wong, W. and Terrault, N. (2005); Zou, S., Forrester, L. and Giulivi, A. (2003).

Law that were elaborated in the introduction; as an expression of hepatitis C as always already multiple. But making this connection in any meaningful way, and to any useful purpose, entails taking a series of steps. Below we systematically engage the medical notion of quasispecies with Mol and Law's observations about complexity to draw together a feminist quasispecies epistemology. In doing so, we also attend to recent feminist engagements with notions of materiality which argue that the material needs to be brought back into critical accounts of the social (Barad 1998; 2001; 2007). We will then take this epistemology to the literature to see what it brings into view about the medical production of disease.

Populations, clans, multiplicity

The hepatitis C virus turns out in the medical literature not to be a virus at all. Instead it is a population of viruses that differ at the level of genotype, subtype and quasispecies.[2] Hepatitis C genotypes can differ in genetic sequence by up to one third. Within each genotype are numerous subtypes, incorporating further variations. Individuals living with the virus can 'host' millions of different quasispecies, or genetic forms of the virus that differ further due to changes occurring during replication within the body. According to an authoritative factsheet on hepatitis C (Franciscus 2010: 1):

> hepatitis C constantly changes and mutates as it replicates – more than 1 trillion hepatitis C virions replicate each day. During the replication process, the hepatitis C virus will make 'bad' copies or errors in the genetic make-up of the newly replicated viruses.

When the body in which the virus is reproducing generates an effective immune response to the most common (or 'master') quasispecies, this quasispecies is destroyed, leaving other quasispecies to persist and mutate until they too are identified by the immune system and destroyed.

So, hepatitis C changes constantly. It reproduces itself, but in so doing, sacrifices itself to new forms of self. These new forms are the result of errors – of incompetence, haste, sheer volume. Yet, as the factsheet also tells us (Franciscus 2010: 1):

> The process of constant mutation helps the virus escape the body's immune response – when the dominant quasispecies is eradicated, another quasispecies emerges.

---

2   The term quasispecies was first coined in research published in 1977. It was used to describe certain ensembles of variant reproductive molecules, and was not directly related to hepatitis C (as is evident in the date of the research). See Más et al. (2010) for a summary of this research.

It seems hepatitis C's orientation to error is also its strength. Martell et al. noted this in 1992 (3225): 'This quasispecies model of mixed RNA virus populations implies a significant adaptation advantage'. They went on to explain that this 'allows for the rapid selection of the mutant(s) with better fitness for any new environmental condition', but also note that 'quasispecies will remain in stable equilibrium with little evolution of its consensus or master sequence as long as conditions are unchanged'. Much more recently, Bowen and Walker (2005: 415) point, with some awe, to hepatitis C's relative genomic 'simplicity' that nevertheless allows for complex changes during replication. The proneness to error in hepatitis C, they note, 'is intrinsic to its persistence, allowing for rapid evolution to adapt to immune selective pressure exerted by the host'.

Host? Discussion of the virus 'host' appears intermittently in material on hepatitis C quasispecies, and in the broader review and summary literature traced here. The role of the host in shaping the virus is often alluded to, but not treated in any depth. Yet this role appears to be significant. As Davis explained in 1999 (245), 'The diversity of quasispecies in any individual is related to the size of the individual inoculum. However, the evolution of quasispecies from a common inoculum varies with the host'. In other words, two individuals infected with the same sample of hepatitis C positive blood would, over time, generate significantly different ranges of quasispecies in their bodies. These ranges are dependent upon 'environmental' factors experienced by the virus, that is, on individual differences in each body. In short the genetic makeup of the virus actually undergoes change in its involvement with its environment. This is accounted for in the literature in conventional evolutionary terms: the virus reproduces rapidly, and the errors introduced during this rapid reproduction are either advantageous or disadvantageous. Those that work with the environment best persist. Those that do not die out.

While the literature regularly attributes disease chronicity (and in this sense, the 'success' of the virus) to the instability of the virus, doubts about these assumptions are also regularly raised in the literature across time. For example, debate has continued over whether hepatitis C's tendency to produce quasispecies causes the disease's persistence in the body, or whether the persistent nature of hepatitis C allows for the production of more quasispecies (Alter 1991: 644). Taking a different tack, Smith et al. (1997: 1511) noted in 1997 that aspects of genotyping technique (PCR amplification via reverse transcription) and broader research method were crude enough to warrant suspicion that research may be magnifying the role of quasispecies in interpretations of hepatitis C's persistence.

Other confusions occur in relation to some of the most basic aspects of the debate. If hepatitis C is multiple, so is the language used to discuss it. Smith et al. (1997: 1511) note in this context that even the word 'quasispecies' has multiple lives. It is, for example, used to refer to each of the virus sequences that comprise the collection of quasispecies, or to the unrelated species variants within one individual but arising from different sources, or to several other phenomena. This variation is in part a product of the highly volatile nature of knowledge about hepatitis C since its naming.

The relationship between genotype, subtype and quasispecies differences and practical issues such as symptoms, disease progression and treatment efficacy also continues to be the subject of research and debate, but some certainties have solidified over time within the literature. Some genotypes are, for example, considered more harmful to the body than others. Some are more easily treated, that is they are more likely to be cleared from the body by treatment with combination interferon and ribavirin drug therapy. The significance of subtypes is less clear. Some argue subtypes impact on treatment outcomes, the natural history of disease and the success of transplants, and there is speculation that subtypes will be more closely considered in determining treatment dosage and duration in future. Thus, in spite of the articulation of some certainties about the disease, the characterisation of hepatitis C within medical discourse remains volatile. This is not to say, of course, that this volatility is thoroughly or explicitly articulated in the literature examined here. More will be said about this later. In the meantime it is enough to note that the discourse of knowledge production deployed within the material is relentlessly forward-looking in tone, and as such, rarely acknowledges or reflects on medicine as having been mistaken or wrong in its past pronouncements.

In all, it is possible to speak of hepatitis C as embracing, or better, comprising, a range of uncertainties, populations or clans. Medical knowledge is volatile and multiple, as is the terminology and even the virus 'itself'. The relationships between various putatively separate phenomena are unclear, or, we might say, difficult to sustain under analysis. Cause and effect cannot be straightforwardly distinguished. Genome and environment are mutually dependent. Knowledge and method shape each other.

Building on the discussion of complexity offered in the Introduction, we can make a series of connections between the idea of quasispecies and theorisations of method inspired by contemporary feminist and science studies. Mol and Law suggest we can generate accounts of complexity when we acknowledge that phenomena are always 'more than one and less than many' (2002: 11); when we refuse the temptation to produce reductive and totalising overviews. Hepatitis C is an especially compelling instantiation of this idea in that it is both clearly acknowledged as multiple, and also actively, some would say, aggressively 'held together' as a phenomenon for purposes that can (and later will) be argued to be principally political.

Where phenomena are recognised as multiple, it is necessary to adopt strategies for their discussion in ambitious social science research such as that undertaken in this book that can to some degree accommodate, or let us say enact, this multiplicity. For example, according to Mol and Law, we must try to avoid polarising chaos and order, and we must necessarily treat material phenomena as emergent within rather than anterior to the social. Clearly, the quasispecies account of hepatitis C can be read in this light. As we have been told, the disease is always already

multiple. Its essence is always in motion via mutation. Indeed 'chaos', in the form
of continual error, is both its defining nature and its means of survival and success.
Causation is also complicated here. Do quasispecies precede persistence or follow
it? Does it, in any case, make sense to separate these two factors? Knowledge
production about hepatitis C does not rest, nor does the genome – it is continually
in flux. The environment within which the genome 'evolves' must also constantly
change in that it is a human body. Indeed, the way the body is enrolled in medical
advice about responding to hepatitis C suggests that diagnosis with the disease
will at least sometimes generate active efforts on the part of the patient to change
this environment through injunctions against drinking, and in favour of 'healthy
lifestyle choices' such as good diet and exercise. For our purposes here we shall,
therefore, nominate the following features of a quasispecies epistemology:

1. Constant motion;
2. Repetition and change through error;
3. Error and chaos as productive – as enfolded in, rather than antithetical to,
   order;
4. Phenomena as always already more than one and less than many;
5. Causation as multidirectional, non-linear;
6. Contingency of sameness and difference.

Of course, a key element of a quasispecies epistemology informed by the work of
Mol and Law must be a reconsideration of ontology beyond positivist accounts
offered within science in general and medical discourse in particular. While the
analysis being developed here is provoked by medicine's presentation of the
hepatitis C virus as always changing, multiple, uncertain and so on in its materiality,
our treatment of these characteristics is not a positivist one. In other words, as
should be evident in what has been said thus far, the epistemology developed
here has not been generated via the assumption, as made in the article by Bowen
and Walker (2005) and in other work cited above, that hepatitis C is an *a priori*
material object with essential or intrinsic attributes to be taken for granted. That is,
whereas Martell et al. (1992: 415) explain that the proneness to error in hepatitis
C, 'is intrinsic to its persistence, allowing for rapid evolution to adapt to immune
selective pressure exerted by the host', the epistemology posited here would not
take for granted as separate from and anterior to knowledge production either the
phenomenon that 'persists' (the virus) or the phenomenon that 'hosts' (the body).

　　Instead, in keeping with feminist science studies work such as that of Barad
and Haraway and science and technology studies work such as that of Latour, Mol
and Law this approach takes materiality as emergent; as the product and producer
of ontological politics. This book's first author (Suzanne Fraser) has spelt out this
approach to materiality elsewhere in an engagement with Karen Barad's 'agential
realism' (Fraser and valentine 2008), and the analysis offered here should be read

as in keeping with this approach.[3] Most importantly, an approach to the materiality of hepatitis C that treats it as emergent allows us to engage with disease as a thoroughly political object, the attributes and effects of which are radically open to change. In the next three sections we track a key theme that runs through the articles – that of scientific progress – mapping, or perhaps 'walking' as Law and Mol would suggest (2002), how discussions of the knowability and containability of the disease, the framing of transmission and the action of testing have changed, and thinking through the meaning and effects of these changes. All of these themes shape each other, but will be discussed separately here as a means of drawing out their specific effects and implications as well as their relationships.

Holding progress together

Tracking reviews of scientific knowledge on disease across time offers fascinating though partial insights into the constitution of scientific progress itself. The reviews analysed here appeared on an irregular basis, cover a variety of topic areas within the field of hepatitis C research and often leave large gaps in their accounts of knowledge development. For these reasons, they do not together provide an especially seamless overview of change over time. Of course, as Mol and Law have suggested, seamless overviews come at a price. In bringing together bits and pieces of thought and observation, they create coherence, thereby constituting the objects and subjects they seek to describe, but also excluding or othering elements that do not apparently fit. These elements can continue to haunt the newly constituted object, disrupting it, reminding us that all is not as it seems. Where the constituted object fails to lend itself effectively to conventional explanations, such as in those cases where disadvantage or inequity is insufficiently well articulated, this exclusion and haunting emerges as a significant impediment to understanding and effective action. The result, were we to attempt such a process of constitution here, would be something akin to the timelines often constructed in attempts to track medical knowledge over time, and of which hepatitis C has attracted many (see for example Nature Reviews (Microbiology) at http://www.nature.com/nrmicro/journal/v5/n6/fig_tab/nrmicro1645_I1.html and BBC News at http://news.bbc.co.uk/2/hi/uk_news/scotland/988329.stm). Timelines carry within them a temporal logic that tends to posit states of lesser development moving to states of greater development, as the 'truth' of objects is gradually revealed. The reviews found in the peer-reviewed medical literature to do the same – both individually and collectively – if we allow them to. By this we mean that a discursive strategy consistently found in the material, one it is wise to register and query, is the positing of breakthroughs, advances and achievements. It is also the case that obstacles and challenges are identified, but as we will show below, the language of the obstacle

---

3   At least insofar as this is evident to the authors.

or the challenge reinforces, rather than departs from, the generally progressivist, triumphalist tone.

The first review of knowledge (Alter 1991) appears shortly after the hepatitis C genome had been cloned and sequenced. This event forms the basis for many expressions of medical triumph over time in the literature, but it most directly anchors the positive tone of material contemporaneous to it. So, as Alter (1991: 648) puts it, 'There is optimism that a recombinant vaccine could be produced because the entire genome has been sequenced'. Alter describes vaccine development as in its 'infancy', a metaphor that acknowledges an absence of expertise but also implies that, just as infants grow and mature, so will knowledge. Alter also states (1991: 649) that '[t]he cloning of HCV is a remarkable accomplishment that has led to many important observations in a very short time. Our knowledge is expanding exponentially...'.

Reference to the early discoveries and triumphs of hepatitis C scientific research is made over and over in this literature, even, or especially, as realisations about the disappointing prospects for achieving in a timely fashion key goals such as a vaccine began to sink in. Three years after Alter's comments, for example, Purcell (1994: 181) describes the cloning and sequencing of the hepatitis C virus as 'one of the outstanding scientific achievements of the past decade'. This does not mean all is solved however. While, according to Purcell, the near-eradication of iatrogenic transmission of hepatitis C via blood products (such as those required in surgical operations or consumed by people with haemophilia and thalassaemia) has been 'nothing less than spectacular', the control of what originally was called 'community acquired' hepatitis C (more on the demise of this term later) is billed as a 'major challenge'. Here is our first opportunity to consider the language of challenge in the context of scientific research.

Given that Purcell also states that (1994: 181) 'The rapid rate of progress since 1989 is evidence that the foundation for understanding HCV was in place and ready for the inevitable breakthrough', we can surmise that he is confident and optimistic about continued growth in knowledge in the area. Where breakthroughs are inevitable, challenges, it would seem, are surmountable. Indeed, in popular usage, the word 'challenge' usually refers to positive phenomena that generate new thought and practice, and almost always lead to resolution and concomitant progress. Admittedly, Purcell does not altogether avoid the alternative language of failure. As he also argues (1994: 185), 'The failure of the scientific community to develop a specific serological test for NANB hepatitis led many to think of applying the recently discovered methods of recombinant DNA technology...'. Yet even here, a progressivist teleology is applied. By virtue of this initial failure, and the turn to recombinant techniques, a major global scientific achievement was generated: the cloning of the hepatitis C genome. Thus, failure is productive, a precursor to success.

Indeed, progressivist language saturates the material. The repeated use of terms such as 'infancy', 'evolution', 'promise' and 'horizon' in reviews across the 1990s instantiates a logic of inevitable forward movement in knowledge. Of course, the hindsight afforded by our analysis at this point in time allows the recognition that many cases of optimism were misplaced. So, for example, by 1999 Walker (520) notes that 'several promising opportunities for drug development have already been discovered through molecular biology'. Further, according to Walker (1999: 528), 'it appears that an effective anti-HCV treatment will emerge in the next ten years'. How accurate has this prediction proven to be? Perhaps an assessment hangs on the meaning of the word 'effective'. In 1997 Lindsay noted the prospect of improved treatment via the introduction of combination interferon and ribavirin treatment, a development that did turn an entirely ineffective form of treatment into something having some useful effect for a minority of treated patients. And later, pegylation again improved clearance (ovcure) rates in treatment. Yet, even in 2010 treatment outcomes remain uncertain, and the treatment regime remains punishing and out of reach for the majority of people living with hepatitis C (See page 85 for details on the effects of the treatment). The extent to which the prediction of treatment effectiveness can be judged accurate is, in this sense, necessarily subjective. Certainly, by most measures, long term, heavily incapacitating treatment that is unsuccessful in between 20 and 50 per cent of patients would not be considered outstanding, spectacular or a remarkable accomplishment.

Given early disappointments, the material covering the decade from the year 2000 would be expected to be rather more sober in tone than that sourced from the earlier period. Some sobriety is indeed evident here and there. Sarbah and Younossi's piece, for instance, concedes that (2000: 136), 'current interferon-based regimens for the treatment of HCV, even in the eyes of the optimist, are woefully inadequate'. Directly following this concession, however, Sarbah and Younossi conclude with an unequivocal re-affirmation of the scientific research process, couched in the familiar terms of the scientific quest: 'Thus the search continues...'. In 2001, Bonkovsky echoes earlier congratulatory reflexes by retelling the narrative of the sequencing of the hepatitis C genome, describing it as a (2001: 612), 'triumph of modern molecular biology and recombinant DNA techniques'. But Bonkovsky's account is not entirely positive either. He too notes problems in the progression of knowledge, observing that difficulties in diagnosing hepatitis C mean knowledge about natural history has been 'confounded' by a lack of information about date and duration of infection (2001: 621). He also notes that treatment is 'not particularly efficacious' (2001: 637). As in the many other cases that consistently revert to optimism, this view is qualified by the observation that (2001: 641), 'interferon and/or ribavirin have anti-inflammatory and antifibrotic effects on the liver even when they are not able to eradicate HCV'. In other words, treatment failure can also be reclassified as success depending on how success is defined, that is, if existing understandings among patients of the goal of treatment as clearance are shifted or dispensed with. By 2005, one review (Fung and Lok 2005: 300) is asserting the 'impressive gains ... in the treatment of ... infection in hard-to-treat patients', and another (Wong and Terrault 2005: 507) describing the past decade as having 'seen substantial improvement' in treatment. This piece also acknowledges the limitations of current therapy, arguing that (2005: 517) 'problems with tolerability and efficacy should be met by increasing enrolment of previously excluded groups in treatment: those with HIV, those with a mental illness, and those on opioid pharmacotherapy treatment for heroin addiction'. The rationale for this appears to be the need to include as many people as possible able to tolerate the existing treatment regime, given alternatives are (2005: 517), 'at least 3-5 years away from approval'. Here, scientific failure gives rise to a certain kind of benefit: increased access to treatment, albeit treatment that has been deemed of poor quality.

How should we view the literature's narratives of success from success, success in spite of disappointment and success from outright failure, in relation to Law and Mol's observations about method, and our own attempts to 'walk' a quasispecies epistemology? As the figure of the walk, with its emphasis on partiality, would suggest, this epistemology and its recognition of the productivity of error is not intended as a tool for reframing ragged and multiple events into seamless teleological tales of triumph. Instead, it should be mobilised to aid us in linking into our analysis those elements often left absent in accounts of change obsessed with the present-as-end-point or culmination: the dead ends, the hiatuses, the points at which conventional narrative simply peters out and cannot be sustained – those elements usually actively or unknowingly 'othered' in accounts of knowledge and practice. An important observation to be made in this context, that is, where an effort is made to notice the othered (Law 2004), is the inconsistency in the language of success and progress applied in this literature. Most obvious when the uncertainties of treatment outcome are broached, this inconsistency can be identified in the application of the notion of 'failure' to patients. So, for example, Fung and Lok (2004: 304) discuss treatment of acute hepatitis C, advocating 'close monitoring of patients with acute HCV and treatment of those who fail to clear the infection spontaneously after 3-6 months'. Likewise, Pearlman argues that (2004b: 344): 'If certain patients fail to achieve a 12-week treatment milestone, an early virological response, they [should] be taken off treatment early, potentially sparing them from unnecessary medication'. Thus, while scientific accounts of scientific responses to hepatitis C consistently turn away from the idea of failure and towards that of success even where progress is disappointing or absent, these same accounts often unequivocally mobilise notions of failure elsewhere, even against the intended beneficiaries of scientific progress: medical patients. It is, on the face of it, ironic that while medicine is consistently described as at least on its way to achieving success, patients for whom medicine can yet do nothing, or whose medicine does not actually work, are themselves described as having failed. Yet this kind of distribution of effects has a clear function: where an epistemology of progress is adhered to, and the chaotic, multiple and partial are repressed, the boundaries of scientific endeavour are aggressively demarcated, allowing chosen elements left within these boundaries to be seen as actually or imminently successful, and expelling other elements so as to limit their disruptive significance. This epistemology of the unitary, bounded, coherent and progressive generates outliers, the abject and the stigmatised. It is this that a quasispecies epistemology, inspired both by theory and by the materiality of the virus itself, aims to disrupt.

Testing knowledge

The phenomena that become framed as failures are instructive. Another example can be found in the discussion of hepatitis C testing, in which technologies of testing emerge as central to understandings of the disease, its modes of transmission, its natural history and the rate at which spontaneous clearing (or 'successful clearing' in the terms elaborated above) takes place. Indeed, a primary thread throughout the literature is the development of, and continual quest for, effective reliable tests for hepatitis C. In 1991, Alter notes, for instance, that available antibody tests produce diagnoses that account for no more than 80 per cent of non-A, non-B cases (and often less), and that this is likely to change when testing becomes more sensitive. Alter also posits the possibility of two diseases comprising the non-A, non-B category – a form that produces chronic hepatitis C and another that produces a quickly cleared infection. Ultimately Alter favours the test insensitivity argument in this debate, but provides no clear evidence for this preference. It is a choice borne out in later accounts which do indeed retain a single disease entity (see Chapter 2 for more on the singularisation of hepatitis C). Alter's views on a second key issue in the development of knowledge – the sexual transmission of the disease – are, however, rather less confident. He concludes from mixed data that sexual transmission is likely, but argues that rates are probably low. Definitions of 'sexual transmission' are of course important here, but more recent accounts of the disease no longer frame it in this language. Instead it is seen as blood-borne, with some blood-to-blood contact possible during sexual intercourse. The significance of this distinction is not always made clear, however. What is sexual transmission really? Is sexual activity related to blood exposure properly classified as sexual transmission or as blood-borne transmission? As with many aspects of the disease, a lack of clarity surrounding sexual transmission persists (Lenton et al., 2011).

Likewise, with testing, although health promotion materials and other sources of information about hepatitis C regularly depict diagnosis as straightforward and unequivocal, this is, to date, far from the case. The complexity involved in producing a reliable diagnosis of hepatitis C infection can be read from the range and sequencing of testing currently in place. At present, testing for hepatitis C entails the following procedures:

1. Hepatitis C antibody test, which looks for antibodies to the hepatitis C virus in the blood. This test indicates that the patient has at some time been exposed to the virus;
2. Hepatitis C polymerase chain reaction (PCR) tests, which are usually conducted after the antibody test. They look for the virus itself in the

blood (rather than the antibodies produced in response to the virus). In part they confirm the disease is still active and has not been cleared. There are three such tests: one to detect the presence of the virus, one to estimate the amount of virus in the blood (viral load) and one to determine the specific genotype of the virus;

3. Liver function test, which provides information on the extent to which the liver is functioning normally. This test is conducted once activity has been established and information about the condition of the liver is sought. It looks for levels of alanine aminotransferase (ALT). If levels are above pre-established norms, liver damage is likely;

4. Liver biopsy, an invasive test in which a small section of the liver is removed and analysed to establish whether and to what extent the liver has been affected by the presence of hepatitis C. It looks for scar tissue in the liver, taken to indicate cirrhosis or fibrosis;

5. Fibroscan, a test conducted by ultrasound. It too looks for scar tissue, and in some cases can replace the painful and invasive biopsy.

Beyond these core tests, other tests are also either in development or only occasionally used. So, for example, some researchers seeking to understand better the behavioural factors behind some individuals' apparent protection from hepatitis C use the more rarely used 'Elispot' test. One study found as a result of this specific testing strategy that previous assumptions about hepatitis C exposure and risk behaviour could not be sustained. The different testing regime revealed greater rates of hepatitis C exposure than previously thought (Hellard et al. 2010):

> Elispot testing showed over a third of participants lacking anti-HCV antibody and HCV RNA had been exposed to the virus. This result shows that all previous epidemiological studies of HCV in IDUs suffer from misclassification bias: attempts to quantify relationships between behavioural and other characteristics associated with HCV exposure – on the basis of anti-HCV antibody and/or RNA – are flawed. The behaviour of the persistently HCV Elispot-negative participants was no different to that of participants who became HCV Elispot or RNA-positive, leaving open the possibility that these few participants have superior immune function that protects them from infection.

Viewed from the perspective of the quasispecies epistemology, we can see how knowledge about, and practices of, hepatitis C testing (and thus of research and prevention) have been in constant motion since the naming of the disease and earlier. Further, the technological limitations of testing mean that we can say the disease has been profoundly constituted through a series of errors. This process of constitution cannot merely be dismissed as misguided; as something that can simply be abandoned. The knowledge it produced shaped the epidemic by shaping public health and other responses to it. We need to consider, for example, the potential impact on public health responses to forms of hepatitis C testing that produce high levels of false negatives and an understanding of transmission that left up to 40 per cent of non-A, non-B hepatitis unaccounted for. One possible result might have been the design of responses not effectively targeted to the most common form of transmission (injecting drug use), thereby allowing infections among people who inject drugs to rise. In this sense, the epidemic has been shaped by the state of knowledge about testing and the processes of testing themselves. To put this differently, testing can be seen to produce different epidemics. Depending on the particular testing regimes in place in different times and places, multiple, differently constituted but interrelated epidemics can be mapped. By this we mean that variations in testing can produce different disease profiles in different regions or demographic areas, leading to speculation or hypotheses about those areas and the reasons for these putative variations (for related discussions of the production of epidemics, see Rosenberg 1992; Aronowitz 1998). In turn, public health responses specific to these 'different epidemics' can emerge, shaping these epidemics as they do.

An additional way in which testing can be seen to shape hepatitis C epidemics can be found in the deployment of testing based on existing assumptions about risk and prevalence. For example, in 2000 Sarbah and Younossi stated that, in relation to 3rd generation assays:

> despite the high sensitivity and good positive predictive value (90%-95%) of these tests in a high risk population (e.g. setting of abnormal liver enzyme tests and history of prior intravenous drug abuse), with low-risk populations (e.g. volunteer blood donors) the positive predictive value is reduced and confirmatory tests are helpful (2000: 128).

Sarbah and Younossi's point is that where liver problems are identified or a history of injecting drug use has been acknowledged, a positive assay is sufficient proof of infection. Where a blood donor does not have relevant signs of liver trouble or does not acknowledge past or present injecting drug use, a positive assay result should not be taken at face value. Given the stigmatised status of injecting drug use, and the widespread reluctance to reveal past or present injecting, it is surprising to find skepticism about positive status constituted in these terms. Sarbah and Younossi insist that (2000: 129), 'In view of the assortment of available diagnostic tests for HCV, a rational approach to testing is needed', yet what might constitute the most 'rational' set of assumptions and therefore actions emerges as profoundly, and not necessarily desirably, intuitive.

Assigning mystery

Given the vagaries of knowledge about hepatitis C, and the extent to which concrete action has been premised on information later explicitly challenged and assumptions (such as the nature of injecting drug use and the characteristics of those people engaging in it) that are profoundly socially and culturally produced, it is perhaps unsurprising that metaphors of mystery and elusiveness appear continually in the literature. As in the case we described earlier of the assignment of failure to patients rather than to medical treatment, mystery, uncertainty and even 'insidiousness' are usually located outside scientific practice by positioning them explicitly in the virus. Sometimes grammar even locates them within the body of the patient. Rarely, if ever, are the limits or functions of medicine or broader scientific practice constructed as the cause or locus of uncertainty or mystery.

To return to the first published review of knowledge (Alter 1991: 644), for instance, we read: 'the agent [virus] eluded serological detection for more than a decade'. In 1994 (181), Purcell describes the disease as having moved from a 'shadowy enigma' to an 'important public health problem' and in 1997 (12S) he says that the significance of the variability of the hepatitis C genome 'remains elusive'. In 2000 Sarbah and Younossi (125) describe hepatitis C as an 'insidious disease', 'silent' and 'smoldering'. This language of insidiousness, elusiveness and mystery can be found consistently throughout the literature, so that by 2007 (601), Perez still refers to disease 'mysteries', although in this case these are the 'mysteries of viral hepatitis' as a whole, rather than hepatitis C alone. In Perez's view, the number of viral hepatitis mysteries 'disentangled' in the preceding 50 years is 'gratifying'.

Beyond the use of the pejorative terminology of insidiousness to describe the nature of the virus action in the body, many other vividly negative terms and figures of speech are used. Bhandari and Wright (1995, 309), for example, use conventional, if extremely negatively loaded, medical terminology in describing hepatitis C as 'indolent'. Likewise, Walsh and Alexander (2001: 501) describes the absence of symptoms in some hepatitis C positive people as 'sinister' in that it allows undetected disease progression. Other constructions in the literature produce notable confusions of agency. Bhandari and Wright (1995: 3012) for example, explain that '[a]pproximately 60-80% of patients infected with HCV following transfusion insidiously develop chronic hepatitis and cirrhosis'. Here, patient rather than virus behaves in an insidious fashion. In the same way, Hwang (2001: 230) states that 'patients ... often progress to cirrhosis insidiously'.

All these language devices stand out in the literature in that they so clearly depart from ideals of purely rational and unemotional scientific discourse. It would be tempting at this point to speculate that the language choices found here somehow reflect pre-existing stigmatising attitudes towards the population most heavily affected by hepatitis C – people who inject drugs. This interpretation would, of course, be ahistorical, in that many of the expressions appear before clarity emerged about which groups are indeed most closely associated with the epidemic. This does not mean there are no examples of changes in language that can be speculatively attached to issues of stigma however. Perhaps the most obvious is the early circulation of the expression 'community-acquired' to describe hepatitis C transmission that did not occur as a result of blood transfusion, but instead was passed from individual to individual socially. In the body of literature analysed here, this term drops out of use as recognition that most 'community'-based transmission occurs via the sharing of injecting equipment used for the consumption of illicit drugs. Including injecting drug use and the people engaged in it within definitions of the community seems to be actively avoided here. In this case it is less easy to dismiss the impression that language in the scientific literature has been influenced by social values. A contrary case that nevertheless serves to support this point can be found in recent literature on the acquisition of hepatitis C in Egypt, a country heavily affected by the disease due to a history of widespread non-sterile population-level vaccination practice. Thus, one 2010 article (Saleh et al.) discussing hepatitis C positive Egyptian children is titled 'Incidence and risk factors for community-acquired hepatitis C infection from birth to 5 years of age in rural Egyptian children'.

Operating at a more subtle level in the language of mystery surrounding hepatitis C are the notions of silence that can also be found in the material. Here it is useful to consider some of Law's observations about research method and silence. We will then turn to specific examples of this language and consider them alongside what we already know about the history of testing and diagnosis for hepatitis C. In his book on social science method, *After Method: Mess in Social Science Research* (2004), Law talks explicitly about the nature of silence. As with some of the work on which he has collaborated with Annemarie Mol, this discussion is concerned with the need to juggle complexity and simplification in research. One of the ways in which this juggling must be managed, he argues, is via the creation of silence. So, in his view, all methods (2004: 107) 'make silences and non-realities as well as signals and realities'. How are realities made? Law points to the distinctions that are routinely made between 'right' and 'wrong' patterns of similarity and difference when phenomena are being investigated. Which apparent similarities matter in best understanding an object, practice or other phenomenon? Which apparent differences? Which do not? In conducting research, or producing knowledge in other ways, choices must be continually made about the similarities and differences – the patterns – that should be focused on and articulated. As these choices are made, and the observer/researcher/participant throws her or his lot in with a particular set of assumptions and patterns, other assumptions and patterns that might also have been chosen, observed and recorded, are consigned to silence. As Law puts it (2004: 110), 'silence and non-realities are also artful effects'. In generating accounts of what Law calls 'out-thereness' (this term being an attempt to engage what is usually, and too statically, thought of as 'reality'), we are always already involved in mutually dependent processes of silencing and amplification.

By amplification Law means the processes by which researchers (or anyone creating knowledge and thus reality) choose patterns of interpretation to pursue in their 'data'. When we observe, he says, we seek patterns, and the patterns we come to see as early glimmers, are then built upon by further selective attention. This selective attention then produces new corroborating data. In other words, as

Law says of a research project he conducted and the process of data analysis he undertook (2004: 111):

> The signal grew against a growing background of silence. Indeed, in due course I found it difficult to attend to forms of talk which did not fit this basic pattern of repetition.

Here we would question Law's use of the expression 'background' to describe the constitutive other to signal. It is clear from Law's argument that silencing processes constitute realities rather than merely producing a seemingly passive backdrop to them. There is much else here, however, that resonates with the processes and implications entailed in hepatitis C testing and subsequent understandings of the disease. When Law goes on to range 'science' alongside 'silence' as a means of spelling out that method assemblages unmake and disallow many more realities than they produce, our thoughts turn to testing and diagnosis. He goes on to insist that (2004: 118) 'the disciplines that are currently pressed upon us [here he is referring to epistemological approaches developed via Enlightenment notions of reality – scientific method being the core model] tend to make the wrong kinds of silence. They tend to make the silences of Euro-American metaphysics'. This silencing has, it is clear, many costs. Indeed Law asks us to explicitly consider just what phenomena particular methods silence as they produce presence.

Clearly we can take this question up in relation to hepatitis C testing and the knowledge it has produced about the disease – the realities it has materialised. Perhaps most directly, we can understand testing as a mode of 'listening' that in its limitations, and degrees and kinds of sensitivity, also produces silence. Above we argued that testing has the capacity to shape hepatitis C epidemics in at least three ways:

1. Testing can shape public health responses to hepatitis C in particular ways where there are high levels of false negatives and an inability to account for a large minority of non-A, non-B hepatitis transmissions.
2. The specific testing regimes used in different times and places can create particular perceptions of epidemics in that each create different incidence and prevalence rates among different groups. These perceptions can shape public health responses and, in turn, the material scale and nature of these epidemics through the effects of the responses.
3. The deployment of testing regimes based on existing assumptions about risk and prevalence can also shape rates and responses to them.

In all these cases testing acts as a technology of listening and of silencing. Some signals are amplified and some are silenced. As Law argues, this is a necessary process in research of any kind or – as he puts it – in any kind of method assemblage. His point is not that we must eliminate silencing (this would be impossible and leave us without the ability to craft any kind of order from our data). Instead it is to be aware of these processes of amplification and silencing and continually take them into account.

In relation to the medical literature analysed for this chapter we can make two points based on Law's argument. The first is the perhaps unsurprising observation that the literature does not do as Law suggests. The role of testing, or indeed of any aspect of scientific method assemblage, is not conceived in terms of the signals it amplifies and silences it produces. In keeping with the literature's tendency to rely on a progress model, it often overlooks the silencing role of testing and comprehends changes in testing regimes simply as producing increasingly better methods of listening to signals. So, for example, when Alter (1991: 644) observes that 'The agent [virus] eluded serological detection for more than a decade', we can see that the process envisaged is purely one of increasing insight into *a priori* signals, absent of any perception that in 'detecting' the virus in a particular way, other possibilities simultaneously elude detection, or are silenced.

Notwithstanding this common formulation of scientific knowledge, there are statements to be found in the literature that can be read in line with Law's observations. Thus, Lindsay considers testing for treatment response, warning that (1997: 74S):

> Because of the variability of sensitivity among the PCR-based assays, utility of the data [for establishing treatment response] may be assay specific. Currently, therefore, there is [sic] insufficient data to recommend stopping therapy based on virological testing alone.

Drawing on Law, we can say that Lindsay points to the role of particular method assemblages (different assays) in amplifying certain signals and silencing others. At the same time, however, Lindsay's formulation of the issue adheres quite closely to conventional epistemological commitments in that it implies that, with sufficient data (and presumably with 'better' method assemblages), these uncertainties can be resolved and a single, correct amplification made in which the silencing of relevant realities does not occur. Law, of course, does not argue that amplification and silencing can be refined until the 'correct' reality is revealed. Instead, given that *all* method assemblages are partial and only able to produce their own, idiosyncratic realities, we cannot expect to resolve the nature of reality in this way. Indeed, while Law acknowledges the persistence of 'out-thereness', that which is 'out there' is never treated as single, or as formed prior to the research process. Here Law's epistemology entails ontological commitments also at odds with that of conventional scientific method.

If we look closely at the way testing is articulated in the literature, in particular, at the use of the expression 'sensitivity', this difference becomes very clear. In many reviews of the development of knowledge about hepatitis C, the notion of sensitivity is mobilised in relation to testing. So, Colquhoun (1996: 20), for example, notes that the accuracy of testing is subject to 'thresholds of sensitivity'. Likewise, Sarbah and Younossi (2000) explain early testing as follows:

> The first generation EIA tests, the dinosaur of this family, have been available since 1989 ... Despite making a significant impact early on, these tests were fraught with many problems due to poor sensitivity ... and a high rate of false positivity.

In such cases, we can see that 'sensitivity' is a concept that firmly instates a prior reality to which science must listen, and which can be accurately and transparently captured if only testing can be improved, becoming 'sensitive' enough to the nature of this reality.

By the year 2000, after the third generation of assays has been implemented, discussion of the role of testing in the development of knowledge about hepatitis C becomes less common in the literature. This is perhaps because these later tests are perceived to be highly accurate and their potential for interrupting or obfuscating access to reality seen as minimal. This is, of course, a reasonable and widely held approach to hepatitis C testing in particular and the role of scientific method more generally. Yet it is salutary to consider the recent rise of Elispot testing (referred to earlier) in shaping knowledge about the disease. Mobilised as a result of suspicions that what had been accepted as reliable signs of exposure to the disease may in fact be unreliable, the Elispot test is currently reframing understandings of the meaning of immuno-assays that seem to suggest individuals have not been exposed to the disease. In turn, this promises to reshape knowledge about the nature and the scale of hepatitis C epidemics, and throw into question assumptions about who it is that does come to be exposed to the virus and why. In short, the Elispot test reminds us that, despite the tendency at each stage for scientific literature to present knowledge-making as a building process in which one set of facts is built upon by another, a different story is plausible – one in which scientific method assemblages only ever produce temporary and contingent facts, some of which are entirely discarded later for new temporary and contingent facts. Thus, while the notion of sensitivity assumes a prior, stable reality to which we can become more and more sensitive, the history of scientific research can be read instead as a series of method assemblages that produces, and then shapes, realities in particular ways.

The second, perhaps more significant point relates to the language of 'silence' that consistently characterises the literature's depictions of the disease itself and its actions. It is not, after all, as though the literature makes no reference to silence at all. Quite the opposite. The literature regularly deploys many variations on the idea that hepatitis C is in itself 'silent'. Thus, Sarbah and Younossi's (2000) review article is entitled, 'Hepatitis C: An update on the silent epidemic'. Within the article (2000: 125) they pursue this theme of silence, stating that:

Most patients remain asymptomatic despite silent, insidious progression of the disease.

Similarly, Walsh (2001: 501) says that hepatitis C is characterised by a:

high proportion of patients progressing silently to chronic liver disease with the associated risks of developing cirrhosis and hepatocellular carcinoma.

Other reviews also mobilise the idea of a silent disease, often in less direct ways. For instance, Sarrazin (2004: S88) says, 'Due to the lack of typical symptoms diagnosis of acute hepatitis C is rarely established'. In a different case, Pearlman (2004b: 348) discusses liver function test results, saying:

Although most patients with persistently normal levels have mild chronic hepatitis and a markedly lower likelihood of cirrhosis relative to those with elevated levels, some with persistently normal levels have moderate-to-severe hepatitis on biopsy.

In both these examples the notion of the norm arises – the 'typical'; 'normal levels' – that which we might expect to listen fruitfully in accessing the correct reality. In both cases, however, normality proves misleading or irrelevant. In other words, our tendency to listen to those elements we have already established – the normal – leads us to amplify some signals and silence others. Attending to the normal silences the possibility that for some patients disease is indeed present, or progressing. Here the key issue is the tendency to characterise the disease itself as intrinsically silent, when according to Law, we might as easily say that medicine's method assemblages have generated certain silences, amplified other, sometimes unhelpful, signals, then freighted the responsibility for this process over to the disease itself (and as we have seen with the blurring of the notion of insidiousness to include patients) and to those who have the disease. Our analysis leads us to trace the way in which scientific method as a form of listening is understood and the attribute of silence is ascribed, and to reflect on the implications of this ascription.

This is one important issue to consider in response to the presence of these figures of silence in the literature. Another is the question of which preoccupations the tone of frustration evident in the literature about the 'silent' epidemic reveals. What if we were to present a different account of this silence? We could say, for example, that, luckily, hepatitis C is accompanied by few debilitating symptoms for many people, at least for a significant period after infection. We could say that although this means detection is more difficult, it also means better quality of life for many, at least until symptoms do emerge. Until recently when success rates for treatment became reasonable (and certainly during the period in which many of the reviews negatively interpreting 'silence' were published), individual awareness of infection provided few benefits, especially where diagnosis was not supported with sufficient information and discrimination resulted from subsequent disclosure of status (see Hopwood and Treloar 2003). For some people able to sustain the recommended reductions in alcohol consumption and improvements in diet and exercise as a result of diagnosis, disease progression where it would have occurred might have slowed. For those either not advised to undertake these changes, or unwilling or unable to do so, knowledge of infection had little or no positive utility. Certainly, diagnosis can have an effect on transmission rates, potentially reducing them, and this is no small matter. But this is an epidemiological, or public health, benefit rather than one enjoyed by diagnosed persons themselves (Fraser and Moore, 2011). Indeed key effects of diagnosis for individuals would appear to be the conferral of a sense of contamination and stigma (Fraser and Moore, 2011). We are led to wonder, then, not only whether the idea of a silent epidemic is a rather self-serving medical construct that locates problems to do with knowledge of the virus with the disease itself, but also whether the idea of the silent epidemic and the focus on diagnosis it implies serves public health concerns more than those of individual patients.

Conclusion: 'Holding together' science and disease

Scientific discourse on hepatitis C constitutes many phenomena, most of which cannot be canvassed here. This chapter must itself create silences in its own processes of gathering and creating order. For the record, two such phenomena of note are, 1) the boundary between the human and the non-human as enacted through the use of chimpanzees and other primates in research into hepatitis C transmission, natural history and vaccines, and 2) the boundary between innocent and guilty transmission and disease progression – indicated, as noted earlier, in the fate of the term 'community-acquired' in the literature. In both these cases hepatitis C can be analysed as more than one and less than many, just as it can in looking at questions of progress, testing and silence. Indeed both deserve further research. This chapter has explored hepatitis C from the point of view of what we have called a 'quasispecies epistemology'. Generated in an iterative engagement between theory and the materiality of hepatitis C, this epistemology emphasises:

1. Constant motion;
2. Repetition and change through error;
3. Error and chaos as productive – as enfolded in, rather than antithetical to, order;
4. Phenomena as always already more than one and less than many;
5. Causation as multidirectional, non-linear;
6. Contingency of sameness and difference.

Among other things, it has allowed us to recognise the mutually constitutive nature of knowledge about disease and notions of scientific progress, and the way in which preserving the integrity of the latter entails particular discursive formulations of the former, some of which constitute patients as failures. Here we can ask to what extent this kind of formulation is enabled, at least in recent times, by the marginal status of those most commonly infected by hepatitis C – people who inject drugs – and the limits they face in forming the kind of consumer health movement (see Chapter 5 for more on this issue) that has elsewhere challenged marginalising or pathologising medical reflexes.

Our epistemology has also allowed us to analyse testing in a particular way. By reminding us that diseases are multiple and always already constituted by the devices used to observe or measure them – and that change and development occurs through error as much as through success – we can analyse testing as a series of inevitably flawed method assemblages that constantly make and remake the very phenomenon they seek to trace. Here, the feedback loop between object and method assemblage becomes highly visible, and the politics of measurement is exposed. How, why and when testing occurs has a material impact on the shape of the disease. If we are aware of this, we (that is, science and its social counterparts) can make conscious decisions about how we shape the disease through testing. We can intervene politically in disease via what are apparently the most disinterested and utilitarian of mechanisms.

Lastly, at least in relation to the issues explored here, our epistemology allows us to ask questions of presence, absence and silence. Again, as with the discourses constituting testing in the literature, the medical construction of mystery is revealing. Notions of mystery and silence serve to position scientific endeavour as transparently seeking knowledge – as pursuing an *a priori* set of signals which, when properly detected and decoded, will solve the problems of disease. Also revealing is the emphasis on the inconvenience of the silence of hepatitis C (in that, for example, it is often asymptomatic). This sense of silence as troublesome and unsatisfactory here raises questions about the compatibility or unity of scientific and patient priorities. As we have argued, the account of scientific endeavour produced here is highly partial. It ignores the extent to which science is, as Law points out, wrapped up in silence, and the extent, therefore, to which the signals it amplifies can only ever be partial too. As does Law, we recognise that silencing cannot be eradicated from the production of realities via method assemblages: it is, on the contrary, a condition of that process.

So we do not intend here to warn against silencing altogether. Instead, as we noted earlier, we want to highlight the need to remain conscious of the processes, and as far as possible the content and therefore the effects, of our silencing. The chapters that follow this one also themselves enact certain kinds of presence, absence and othering. They do this with our full (if always partially located) awareness. Our goal in making the kinds of silence we do is to invite the benefits of bringing to presence aspects of hepatitis C to date silenced in medical, social science and public discourse. This chapter has brought to presence some key ideas on which the book as a whole will build. These are: the mutual constitution of ideas of disease and ideals of scientific progress, the role of scientific method assemblages in making disease rather than merely reflecting it, and the importance of paying attention to the dynamics and politics of listening and silence. Together they allow us to view the various processes and sites of the production of this disease from the vantage point of a wholly materialist, thoroughly ontic perspective – a vantage point that allows us to take into account the disease as material phenomenon, and at the same time treat disease as open to change.

Chapter 2
How Disease Holds Together: Hepatitis C and Health Promotion

'We are what we repeatedly do. Excellence, then, is not an act, but a habit'.
(Aristotle, quoted in a safer injecting brochure detailing
ways to prevent transmission of hepatitis C).

Annemarie Mol and John Law's work on anaemia opens with the apparently straightforward but simultaneously complex question: 'What is anaemia?' The concern to explore not only how we understand disease, but how materiality emerges and is performed, has been a constant in Mol's recent work, and one that she returns to in her later research into the lower limb condition known as 'atherosclerosis'. In that research, Mol asks: 'what is lower-limb atherosclerosis?' In asking this question, Mol seeks to engage her readers in an intellectual, conceptual, ontological and political exercise, whereby taken-for-granted notions of what atherosclerosis is and how it is 'formed' are systematically challenged and disrupted. She demonstrates, as we have discussed already, that the ontology of disease – like anything else – is wholly political. In this chapter, we follow the lead of both Mol and Law, continuing the exploration inaugurated in our discussion of medical discourse in Chapter 1. Our focus in this chapter is on a set of epistemological and ontological concerns about the constitution of hepatitis C in health promotion. The starting point for this chapter is, following Mol and Law, simply: what *is* hepatitis C? This is an important question, as we shall see, because hepatitis C as 'disease state' is constituted in action.

We consider these questions through an examination of hepatitis C health promotion and safe injecting materials (hereinafter referred to as 'health promotion materials') published in Australia between 1990 and 2009.[1] Although the

---

1 These materials were collected through a request to peak hepatitis C and HIV/AIDS bodies throughout Australia, as well as policy and advocacy groups (such as organisations representing people who inject drugs), health departments in all states and territories of Australia and other relevant organisations. This request yielded a total of 218 distinct documents addressing people living with hepatitis C, those at risk of hepatitis C, and the friends and family of those living with hepatitis C. The documents were copied and stored in an Endnote library, indexed by year and organisation. A thematic analysis of these materials was produced. We did not aim for a comprehensive or generalised account of the content of these materials. Instead, we sought to identify discursive formations and practices in the account of hepatitis C and its subjects in these materials. Our reading of these materials is a form of discourse analysis. According to Deborah Lupton (1992: 145), discourse analysis is: 'composed of two main dimensions: textual and contextual. Textual dimensions are

focus here is on Australian materials, we argue that many of themes, practices and implications that we explore in this chapter are not limited to the Australian context; indeed, they are indicative of tendencies and trends within other Western liberal discursive contexts (such as the United States of America, the United Kingdom and Canada) in which health promotion is a central organising principle. In this regard, the themes – and, perhaps more importantly, the questions – that emerge in this chapter are equally significant and pressing elsewhere. It is important at the outset to say a little about why we have chosen to analyse health promotion materials and how this analysis differs from that in other chapters. This requires us to also say a little about the argument that we develop in this chapter. In its simplest sense, this chapter argues that like medical testing or treatment, health promotion does not simply *represent* hepatitis C; rather, it *makes* it. Health promotion materialises hepatitis C in ways that both replicate its enactment elsewhere, and depart from it. As we will see, health promotion has it own unique history, aims, objectives, epistemology and ontology. Together, these play a vital role in shaping how hepatitis C is *uniquely* constituted in its domain. Although this constitution is connected to its figuration in medical literature, there are many subtle variations and differences – in language, tone, imagery and emphasis. This is because health promotion has a different set of imperatives from vademecum science, and to the function of medical and scientific reviews and accounts of the kind we considered in the previous chapter. Similarly, it has a different set of imperatives from those of self-help literature, which we consider in the next chapter. These differences are usefully illustrated through a brief consideration of the short history of health promotion itself. According to Macdonald and Bunton (1992: 14) the term 'health promotion' first appeared in 1974 when Marc Lalonde (then Canadian Minister for Health) published a landmark paper entitled *A New Perspective on the Health of Canadians*. Lalonde's argument was that improvements in environment and behaviour (or 'lifestyle') could lead to reductions in health problems. Following the publication of the *Lalonde Report*, the Canadian government shifted its health policy emphasis away from the treatment of existing illnesses and towards the prevention of future ones (Macdonald and Bunton 1992: 14). The promotion of 'healthy living' became a central organising principle of Canadian health policy, an approach subsequently

---

those which account for the structures of discourses, while contextual dimensions relate these structural descriptions to various properties of the social, political or cultural context in which they take place'. What specific 'properties' and 'contexts' might be relevant for a reading of hepatitis C materials? The materials we address in this chapter must be understood as produced by and within health promotion. Accordingly, the discursive formation of hepatitis C considered in this chapter constitutes a materialisation of the disease through the aims, objectives, histories and epistemologies of health promotion. These are matters to bear in mind throughout the chapter, and that we address more fully in the conclusion. More information on these methods and documents can be found in Dwyer, Fraser and Treloar (2011).

taken up with enthusiasm elsewhere.[2] In a practical sense, health promotion expresses itself through individualising and responsibilising tendencies, and an emphasis on self-care and care for others. Some of the key features of the health promotion enterprise are: an ethic of individual responsibility for health care, an emphasis on the precautionary principle, on preventative action, and a focus on 'healthy living' (see Bunton, Nettleton and Burrows 1995).

These features of health promotion are especially important for the analysis we undertake in this chapter. As we will argue, hepatitis C is shaped in particular ways in health promotion materials. This constitution cannot be separated out from the history, aims and objectives of health promotion itself. Although there will be overlaps and connections between the analysis in the previous chapter and this one, it is this placement – within the broader history and context of health promotion – that gives hepatitis C its own unique configuration in these specific materials. When we talk about what hepatitis C 'is', in this chapter, therefore, we speak only about how it is constituted in health promotion, and only about how health promotion makes it as 'disease'. In this chapter we argue that health promotion and the 'new public health' are responsibilising in both intention and effect and that this demands that hepatitis C be produced as stable, coherent and singular. We are also particularly concerned to illuminate some of the political and ethical dimensions of this configuration.

As we will see, health promotion materials address a range of questions, issues and presumed audiences. Information is provided on the history and 'discovery' of hepatitis C in 1989; the virus and how it 'operates'; the 'symptoms' associated with hepatitis C; treatment options, objectives, side effects and outcomes (some of these issues are considered more fully in Chapter 5); routes of transmission; methods for preventing transmission; information on the range of possible psychological and emotional dimensions of diagnosis and the lived experience of hepatitis C; advice on sexuality and sexual relationships; and advice on managing other relationships, obligations, finances and employment. These materials are sometimes aimed at particular audiences. A small number, for example, are written specifically for an (Australian) indigenous audience, utilising local dialects and indigenous imagery. Most literature is directed at people who inject drugs, especially those materials documenting routes of transmission, risk and prevention. In this sense, one of the first observations we can make about hepatitis C-related health promotion materials is that they are characterised by variation: multiple messages, audiences, targets and concerns. In what follows, we consider a set of broader concerns about how this variation figures in other ways in these materials and what this means, not just for how the 'disease' is constituted but also for the politics and ethics of its management more broadly.

---

2   The *Lalonde* report is not the sole factor in the establishment of health promotion as a major policy approach, as Galvin (2002) suggests. For a more detailed summary of other factors in the trend towards health promotion, see Macdonald and Bunton (1992).

This chapter is not the first academic work to consider hepatitis C health promotion materials. Researchers have produced a number of critical analyses of such materials to date. Among other things, these analyses have drawn our attention to the ways in which such materials, through describing routes of transmission and recommending forms of behaviour, constitute particular kinds of injecting subjects (Fraser, 2004) and particular understandings of hepatitis C (Treloar and Fraser, 2004; Fraser and Treloar, 2006; Orsini 2002; Dwyer et al., under review; Seear et al., under review). While hepatitis C-related health promotion literature usually lists the many different ways that hepatitis C is thought to be transmitted (including via the sharing of tattoo needles, razors and toothbrushes), most of this literature is aimed at people who inject drugs. In this regard, as Harris (2005) argues, injecting drug use and hepatitis C are regularly 'conflated' in this literature. In this chapter, we draw upon and extend some of these observations through an examination of two apparently opposed phenomena: the constitution of hepatitis C as 'more than one and less than many' (the virus multiple) and the constitution of hepatitis C as a single 'disease' (the virus singular). As we will argue, these renderings of hepatitis C are achieved through depictions of the virus, its subjects (by which we mean people who acquire the virus) and its effects. These renderings matter, as we shall see, for the same reasons that medical renderings matter: because they help to shape its subjects, the materiality of the virus, and the materiality of the 'epidemic'.

More than one and less than many

As we have already noted, Mol and Law's work on multiplicity and ontology is especially useful in considerations of hepatitis C. In this section we explore the particular aspects of their work most relevant for this chapter, returning to the term 'multiplicity'. Annemarie Mol uses the term 'multiplicity' to argue for the presence of many 'coexistences at a single moment' (Mol 2002: 8). The starting point of Mol's work, for our purposes, is in the distinction she draws between 'construction' and 'enactment'. Seeking to move beyond conventional social constructionist accounts of the kind that have been highly influential in medical sociology, Mol writes:

> The term 'construction' was used to get across the view that objects have no fixed and given identities, but gradually come into being. During their unstable childhoods their identities tend to be highly contested, volatile, open to transformation. But once they have grown up objects are taken to be stablilised. (2002: 42)

On the other hand:

> like (human) subjects, (natural) objects are framed as parts of events that occur and plays that are staged. If an object is real this is because it is part of a practice. It is a reality *enacted*. (2002: 44)

Articulated in Mol's work on anaemia (1999) and later, atherosclerosis (2002), this approach shares something with the work of feminist scholars Judith Butler (1990, 1993) and Donna Haraway (1997), in that it emphasises the 'two-way traffic' (Law 2004: 56) between enactment(s) and realit(ies). To this extent discourse is productive of reality and being is neither stable nor fixed. Her ontology, rather, emphasises iteration; reality is thus multiple. To return to the present context, and as we noted in Chapter 1, hepatitis C cannot be taken to be an object possessing stable meanings and attributes. Rather, hepatitis C is always already enacted; it is a practice that must never cease, if the object is to be said to exist. To the extent that hepatitis C is enacted through practices of ceaseless 'crafting' (Law 2004: 56), the 'meaning' of hepatitis C (or what hepatitis C 'is') is never actually closed, nor is it singular. Morover, the notion of reality as ceaselessly crafted and never stable means that it can always be otherwise. As Mol (1999, 2002) and Law (2004) remind us, perspectivalism, conventional method and social constructionism posit a reality that is both stable and fixed as well as singular. Accordingly, projects designed to attend to multiplicity are political and ethical in their orientation because they aim to reveal the limits of constructionism and perspectivalism and the fiction of singularity. As Mol notes, the enactment of atherosclerosis:

> is more than one – but less than many. *The body multiple* is not fragmented. Even if it is multiple, it also hangs together. The question to be asked, then, is how this is achieved.

Claims to singularity are achieved through multiple means, including processes of 'layering', 'submission', 'rationalisation', 'translation' and the adoption/ imposition of 'single narratives'. Practices such as these, to quote Law (2004: 61) 'work to push the possibility of multiplicity off the agenda'. In short, they render objects stable and 'preserve a general commitment to ontological singularity'. This is what Mol and Law call the work of hanging multiplicity together; the effect is that a collection of practices, objects and subjects comes to be constituted as a single disease state. Likewise we can understand hepatitis C as made to 'hang together' through health promotion materials. But what methods are used to do this work? Most importantly, what are the *effects* of this work of simultaneously making hepatitis C 'hang' together and erasing the evidence of its multiplicity? We consider these questions by attending to the processes of inclusion and exclusion, emphasis and de-emphasis and separation and connection that emerge in health promotion materials. In the following sections we consider, first, how hepatitis C emerges as uncertain, irregular, disjointed and multiple in this literature. Secondly, we consider the productive dimensions of these characterisations, through an analysis of the ways in which they are simultaneously reconfigured, erased and/ or reconstituted through the enactment of a single, overarching narrative about the virus, its subjects and objects. Through this work, hepatitis C comes into being as a single, certain, regular, connected and stable 'disease', even while its subjects, symptoms and 'effects' are paradoxically taken to be none of these things. We then consider the material effects of this process of consolidation.

As we have already noted, this chapter draws inspiration from the work of feminist scholars and others who have theorised the relationship between representation, materiality and reality. Much of this work resonates with Mol and Law's work on multiplicity. These analyses are especially useful, however, because of their explicit engagement with the question of what we can make of texts. In this chapter, we will focus in questions of representation, interpretation and communication. How do we approach these representations? This depends, first, on what questions we ask about representation. The kinds of questions we posit about an area of inquiry can themselves be revealing. If we ask, for instance, whether a thing is represented 'accurately', we assume, and thus enact, a single perspective on reality (this much is implied by the form of the inquiry itself – that there is a stable reality that can be represented 'accurately'). The difficulty of knowing which questions to ask, or what are the right questions, is a matter taken up by Gilles Deleuze, who, in drawing upon the work of Henri Bergson, writes:

> A solution always has the truth it deserves according to the problem to which it is a response, and the problem always has the solution it deserves in proportion to its own truth or falsity – in other words, in proportion to its sense. (Deleuze, 1994: 158)

Following Deleuze, we can say the kinds of questions we ask about, in this case, a text, will produce particular – partial – accounts of knowledge, and thus partial realities, with partial solutions. Early work on the media, for example, focused on a limited set of questions that produced a limited account of the relationship between representation and reality. Early feminist critiques of the media, for example, tended to assume a stable reality separable both from the perspectives of readers and from the representations found in texts. Thus, the media were criticised for producing 'unrealistic' images of women. As feminists and others have pointed out however, particularly in the process of criticising science, reality is multiple and always depends on perspective. The question to be asked of textual accounts can no longer be, therefore, 'whose reality should be represented?' As Brunsdon puts it (1988: 149), 'arguing for more realistic images is always an argument for the representation of "your" version of reality'. As feminists have theorised representation further, the emphasis has shifted to understanding texts such as the media *as discourse*, that is, as a conversation operating within institutional and political forces, yet also productive of resistance. In this model, taken from the work of Michel Foucault, reality is the product of discourse. Representation, in this approach, is seen as both the product of, and the creator of realities, including gender, which itself cannot be seen as a fixed, unchanging referent for the media. Thus, contemporary critiques of the media mounted by feminists interested in transformational politics tend to focus more on what the media 'can do' or 'are doing' politically rather than what they are or what they reflect. The question shifts, therefore, from something like 'How accurate are the media's representations of subject "X"?', to 'what does the media do?'. To bring this question together with the one with which we opened this chapter, we can now say that our analysis addresses the questions: What *is* hepatitis C, as 'done' by health promotion materials? What does health promotion do with hepatitis C?

The virus multiple

In the earliest accounts of hepatitis C in this literature the disease figures as multiple, unpredictable, uncertain, irregular and disjointed. Most obviously, hepatitis C is enacted via repeated accounts of what hepatitis 'is'. Take, for example, a 1991 publication from the Hepatitis C Council of New South Wales. Under the heading 'what is viral hepatitis?', the brochure explains that:

- the virus may cause no symptoms or damage at all;
- the virus may cause no liver damage;
- the virus can cause an acute (short-lived) illness;
- sometimes a virus may cause chronic hepatitis;
- if chronic, hepatitis goes on for several years.

Later, in the same brochure, under 'what happens if you contract hepatitis C?', it is suggested: 'Firstly, the infection may not cause any symptoms', although a series of potential symptoms are later listed. Subsequent materials continue this theme of variability, regularly producing lists of the vast range of symptoms a person may encounter and an explanation of their unpredictability. One publication (Hepatitis Australia 2001 Pt 1), states, for instance:

> Most people do not experience any symptoms for the first 10 years or more after their acute infection. Symptoms of chronic infection can range from mild to severe. They can occur continuously or in bouts. The most common symptoms are:
>
> • fatigue or tiredness
> • lethargy
> • nausea and discomfort in the abdominal region
> • feeling ill if you drink alcohol or eat fatty foods
> • depression
>
> This is a general guide only. Your experience with hepatitis C may be different. Remember that you may feel well, but the damage to your liver caused by hepatitis C may still be progressing.

Alongside such accounts, we often see detailed breakdowns of the proportions of people living with hepatitis C who experience some, all or no symptoms across a given timeframe. We also see accounts of the proportions who experience cirrhosis, liver cancer or liver failure. A 2007 brochure produced by Hepatitis Australia, for example, offers an account of the likely distribution of symptoms. Some of the key statistics here suggest that, on average, one in every four persons clears the infection spontaneously within the first year after infection. Of people who do not undergo treatment, 55 per cent develop liver damage after the first 20 years (the figure is the same for the first 40 years). After the first 20 years, 47 per cent develop mild to moderate liver damage, 7 per cent develop cirrhosis and 1 per cent develop liver cancer or experience liver failure. The rates change across time, with the number of people experiencing mild or moderate liver damage decreasing by 16 per cent a full 40 years after infection, so that the likelihood of developing cirrhosis, on the one hand, or liver cancer or failure on the other, rise (20 per cent and 4 per cent, respectively).

So here we have significant variations in symptoms. What might we make of this? Why is variability significant? How does this account of the variability of hepatitis C work to constitute the disease as object? Can we equate this variability with multiplicity? If so, how? Are there a multiplicity of subjects? A multiplicity of viruses? Perhaps the most important observation to make here is that this collection of diverse and inconsistent symptoms is understood not as an indication of the possibility that hepatitis C is something other than a single disease but, rather, that it emerges as a range of possibilities situated within the boundaries of an expected, 'normal', or 'natural' deviation. The significance of this is a matter to which we will return. Important, for now, is the attribution of symptoms to the function of the virus itself. To return to the example from the Hepatitis C Council of New South Wales above, the exact pattern, distribution and severity of symptoms is in every case attributed to the work of the virus ('the *virus* may cause…'). The virus is afforded total agency and in turn is rendered variable in its actions and diverse in its effects. So here is our first example of multiplicity: the virus, in its multiple actions and *effects*.

Depictions of the virus are also located in explanations of the range of modes of transmission, injunctions to safer injecting, other risk reduction strategies and practices, explanations of the role and function of the liver, and depictions of the impact of the hepatitis C virus on the liver. Often the virus is invested with particular qualities, attributes or traits. At times these are articulated explicitly and at other times implied through depictions of the ways in which the virus might be transmitted. Our starting point for this analysis is representations of transmission and the subject. One account from a 1995 brochure (Hepatitis C Victoria), for example, distinguishes between the many ways in which the virus is transmitted. People who inject drugs can acquire the virus through '*sharing* of needles and syringes during injecting drug use', whereas health care workers acquire it through '*contact* with blood' which can 'lead to infection' (our emphasis). The shift in emphasis – from 'sharing' to 'contact' – operates to constitute the first cohort (people who inject drugs) as both active and culpable in their acquisition of the virus, and the second cohort (health care workers) as passive and innocent. In another example (Hepatitis C Victoria 1996) a list of 'at-risk' subjects is included, along with a description of the specific dimensions of their perceived risk: people who inject drugs are at risk through *sharing*, as are people *undergoing* skin penetration procedures (such as tattoos and body piercing), as are people who *received* blood transfusions, as are health care workers who are *exposed* to blood. Here we can say that there is more than one but less than many subjects in the health promotion materials. Firstly, they are 'more than one' because they are delineated and separated out through their risk profiles, as well as in their agency. This delineation is enacted via subtle variations in the degrees of agency afforded to each group of 'at-risk' subjects, with health care workers and blood transfusion recipients constituted as having the least agency in the viral transaction and people who inject drugs the most agency. Secondly, however, they are also 'less than many', in that only a limited number of subject positions are made available through these articulations. These depictions reflect and reproduce a binary logic in which people who inject drugs are positioned as agentive, culpable and responsible for contracting the virus while health care workers and blood transfusion recipients are vulnerable and without culpability. These discursive formations have considerable ethical and political ramifications insofar as they operate to obscure the range of factors that contribute to the acquisition of hepatitis C among people who inject drugs, such as the limited availability of new, sterile needles and ancillary injecting equipment (see also Seear, Fraser and Lenton, 2010; Fraser and Treloar 2006; Duffin 2005). In this way, certain subjects are constituted through these discursive formations. The relation produced between subject and object is also instructive, however, operating to further compose the virus. In this brochure's rendering of the first group (people who inject drugs) as active (through their sharing of needles and syringes), some agency is extended to the virus. The second group, in contrast, merely comes into contact with (or is exposed to) the virus, signalling the possibility that the virus is itself stagnant, inactive, inert. This implies that there is more than one hepatitis C virus, although again, less than many. Each virus has differing and distinct characteristics. So here is a second example of multiplicity in hepatitis C health promotion materials: the virus, in its multiple *formations.* Later we will look more closely at why health promotion might generate this view.

The phenomenon of spontaneous 'clearing' also features regularly in health promotion materials. The term refers to the process whereby some individuals who have tested positive for hepatitis C later clear the virus without having received medical therapy. In one example, spontaneous clearing is explained in this way:

> Research has shown that about 25 per cent of people infected with hepatitis C will clear the virus within two to six months of becoming infected, but continue to carry antibodies to the virus. The other 75 per cent of people who do not clear

the virus will have an ongoing or chronic infection. (Hepatitis Australia 2007
Part 1)

Here, the virus figures as either or both present, absent, or silent, as variable
and as cyclical. A person living with hepatitis C might spontaneously 'clear'
the virus. In some literature, the virus may later reappear. Whether this can be
attributed to a further, subsequent exposure to the virus is increasingly unclear
(Hellard 2010) although it may occur either through subsequent (re)exposure and/
or a spontaneous and unexplained return of the virus, or both (although not at
once). While there is some overlap between these articulations and those of the
variability of symptomatology we can identify some distinctive features. That is,
although the virus figures in health promotion materials as variable in its actions,
it also materialises as unpredictable and arbitrarily operative, through cycles of
emergence, submergence and re-emergence. Here is, therefore, a third instance of
multiplicity: the virus in its multiple *manifestations*.

It is useful at this point to pause and return to the work of Jacalyn Duffin
(2005), whose analysis of hepatitis C was discussed in the introduction. Duffin
also considered the possibility that there is more than one 'form' of hepatitis C. In
her book *Lovers and Livers*, Duffin observes, first, that there are 'two diseases': the
first is associated with 'contaminated' blood transfusions and (in Canada at least)
regularly attracts compensation. The second does not usually attract compensation
and is instead associated with particular types of behaviour: drug use, sex work
and other 'risky' behaviours. For Duffin, these 'two diseases' reflect and reproduce
assumptions about guilt, innocence and responsibility associated with hepatitis
C that have been well documented elsewhere (Fraser 2004; Fraser and Treloar
2006). Secondly, and perhaps more significantly, she highlights some of the ways
in which these distinctions are achieved. As we have noted in other work (Seear,
Fraser and Lenton, 2010) they are actively produced and reproduced in the common
law, especially where iatrogenic acquisition is recognised as a form of 'innocent'
transmission for which compensation might be awarded (through deployment of
the law pertaining to medical negligence). Compensation is one remarkably visible
way in which the binary logic distinguishing 'guilty' and 'innocent' forms of
hepatitis C transmission functions to categorise and constitute 'different' hepatitis
C subjects. This binary logic operates both ethically and politically to position
individuals with hepatitis C acquired through non-iatrogenic means (most notably,
injecting drug use) as irresponsible and unethical subjects, materialising as it does
so stigmatisation and shame (Fraser and Treloar 2006). These two diseases have
ramifications for the materiality of hepatitis C; in particular, Duffin (2005) argues,
the first version of hepatitis C more regularly attracts money for research and
treatment because those so afflicted are considered to be less culpable and more
deserving of support. The second group figure as beyond help and as undeserving
of both compensation and support.

Although Duffin's work (2005) has great analytical, political and ethical
purchase, we seek to move beyond it in several important respects. First, we do

not assume an *a priori* symptomatology associated with the 'two diseases'. Duffin, in contrast, claims (2005: 122-123) that the first type of hepatitis C is 'usually symptomless', whereas the second form of the disease is 'a serious, chronic liver inflammation'. While we do not doubt the possibility of there being a relationship between the symbolic rendering of hepatitis C and its subjects and the materiality of the disease, such a stark division is not supported by evidence of the distribution of the virus across populations. Secondly, our approach exceeds Duffin's because it does not assume that the 'two diseases' are always already present. Thirdly, and most importantly, while we focus, as does Duffin, on the work that is done to enact different kinds of hepatitis Cs in health promotion materials (the multiplicity detailed above) we also explore the work that is done to create an impression of hepatitis C as singular. This impression also has implications for the material constitution of hepatitis C.

The virus singular

Despite the multiplicity of hepatitis C in the health promotion literature, the disease is also enacted as stable and singular. In this section we consider how and why. In so doing, we must consider questions that have also engaged scholars such as Mol and Law about the work involved in moving between multiplicity and singularity. Is singularisation achieved in relation to hepatitis C? If so, *how*? And finally, *why* might this occur? Claims to singularisation are often uneven and inconsistent in health promotion materials, and it is possible to identify more than one virus or perhaps 'two diseases' (Duffin 2005: 122) in discursive formations of hepatitis C. Although understood as 'part' of a set of viruses affecting the liver, hepatitis C is also constituted as distinctive. Indeed, hepatitis C's original name, 'non-A, non-B hepatitis', marked it as related to, but different from, its others. In this sense hepatitis C is constituted in part through reference to what it is not as well as through that which it almost is. Hepatitis C is not, in the main, framed either as a series of diseases or a set of disease states (although it is often referenced as part of a collection of closely related viruses). The key point here is that hepatitis C is mainly represented as a single disease, and that claims are most often made to singularity. Following our earlier observations about representation as enactment (as opposed to mere depiction), we can say that something happens between hepatitis C's representation/constitution as multiple and its representation/constitution as singular. In health promotion materials, hepatitis C moves back and forth, up and down, changing shape and materialising as a single disease. This shift is not necessarily a one-off event, but part of the ceaseless 'crafting' referred to at the outset of this chapter. This crafting is also related to the specific purposes, histories, objectives and aims of health promotion. To return to the questions we considered at the beginning of the chapter, we ask, how is this singularity achieved? How can we understand the means through which the virus multiple 'hangs together' insofar as it is constituted via health promotion materials? And most importantly, what are some of the implications of such processes? That is, what are the effects of the simultaneous 'hanging together' of hepatitis C alongside the erasure of its multiplicity? What processes of inclusion and exclusion, emphasis and de-emphasis and separation and connection can we find? Three examples follow.

1. The act of naming

Most obviously, the performance of hepatitis C as singular occurs through its inauguration in nomenclature. As Law (1999: 11) has pointed out, singularities are in fact 'performed in the act of naming'. Naming is associated with singularity because:

> The act of naming suggests that its centre has been fixed, pinned down, rendered definite. (Law 1999: 2)

So in part the origins of the erasure of multiplicity can be traced back to the early shift in nomenclature, from non-A, non-B hepatitis, to hepatitis C.

2. The absence of a representative case

Somewhat paradoxically, perhaps, singularity is also achieved through what we call *the absence of a representative case*. If we return to our earlier consideration of variability as to symptomatology, one of the most striking aspects of the hepatitis C health promotion materials is their reluctance to outline an 'average' set of symptoms or a 'likely' scenario for someone newly diagnosed with the condition. By this we mean that it is rare to encounter any articulation of that which is most likely to happen to a given individual, or what pattern of symptoms are most likely to emerge *for you*. Indeed, the emphasis is very much on the unpredictability of individual experience, including the possibility that the virus will spontaneously disappear from the system altogether (this is a matter to which we will return). We can learn much about how accounts of symptomatology matter in the constitution of hepatitis through reference to the mathematical rule of standard deviation. This rule, of course, posits that some degree of deviation either above or below a given average for a population or phenomenon is to be expected; it is, in short, within the realms of 'possibility'. It is only when a deviation well exceeds the boundaries of that deemed an acceptable or predictable degree of deviation that questions of accuracy and reliability arise (see, for example, Bland and Altman 1996; Dodge 2003). When this happens, the object in question begins to take a different form and shape; it will be approached differently, called something else or handled in another way. In this sense, the rules of standard deviation rely upon at least a hypothetical 'centre', from which some deviation can be expected. The centre, or representative case, holds the analysis together, so that deviation is re-constituted as no deviation at all, and extreme deviation is constituted as 'other'. Where the account of symptomatology above differs from this principle is in its lack of a representative case (the 'mean' of the mathematical example). This renders no single symptom or collection of symptoms abnormal, unusual or exceptional; instead, they are all, simply, within the scope of what might be expected. This absence of a representative case works, paradoxically, to produce a remarkably broad account of what hepatitis C is and does (or may not do) in any given case. Together with the act of naming, the absence of a representative case effects the singularisation of hepatitis C and the traces of its multiplicity are swept away.

3. The single narrative

Perhaps most strikingly, the claim to singularity of hepatitis C is performed through a distinct, dominant and overarching narrative of the virus. The notion that a 'single narrative' may play a role in constituting an object as singular comes from Mol's work on the possible ways in which difference in disease is regulated. As Law (2004: 60; our emphasis) explains, paraphrasing Mol, a single narrative is one:

> that *smoothly joins together* theories about the aetiology of [disease] with its anatomical, physiological and diagnostic expressions. Expressions that are in turn linked to judgements about the possibility and desirability of particular interventions. The larger narrative, then, *smoothes together a single coherent object that it describes and explains.*

Our first sense of what this 'larger' or 'single' narrative might look like appears in the form of representations of the virus (subject), its 'hosts' (subjects) and its ultimate target, the liver (object). The narrative threads through the hepatitis C health promotion material, moving in and out, up and down, at times present, at others absent. When we locate it, it generates a coherent and consistent account of the 'virus' and the 'disease' in the face of the multiplicity of *effects, formations* and *manifestations* we identified earlier. The thrust of the single narrative is this: the hepatitis C virus is hidden, sneaky, duplicitous, cunning, inconveniently persistent and unpredictable. The virus is shrewd, sly, and crafty. This unpredictability, persistence and craftiness explains the multiplicity of its effects, its differential formations and the array of its manifestations. These notions of the virus (as unpredictable, resilient, sturdy, cunning, persistent and ubiquitous) regularly feature in health promotion materials, both through textual accounts of the virus and in imagery depicting it. As we noted in Chapter 1, this figuring of the virus (as elusive, insidious, and so on) is, unsurprisingly, also present in medical literature.

One early brochure, suggests, for example, that: 'the hepatitis C virus is quite variable; its exact structure varies in different places around the world'. Here, in spite of apparent variability, unpredictability, and geographical and structural changeability, this is all, simply, hepatitis C. Such accounts of the virus must be read alongside others which imply the unpredictability and duplicity of the virus itself. Take this example produced by the Australian Injecting and Illicit Drug Users League (2008/09), which explains how infection occurs:

> The virus must be present in the blood
>
> The virus leaves the body of a person who is infected
>
> The virus must break through the skin barrier and enter the bloodstream of another person.

Another brochure (AIVL, no date) documents some of the 'special features' of the virus:

> Outside the human host, hep C can stay alive for up to four weeks in a stable environment, for example in a used fit or syringe at room temperature.
>
> In theory, microscopic amounts of infected blood on someone's hands could remain infectious for some time.

In yet another account hepatitis C is described as a 'slow moving virus' (Transmission magazine 2008/09). And finally, in a publication from the Queensland Department of Health (2005), hepatitis C is described in this way:

> Hepatitis C is not a disease that causes problems straightaway, but it can creep up on you and make you really ill.

These depictions mirror those in popular writings about hepatitis C, some of which will be analysed in detail in Chapter 3. In *The Hepatitis C Help Book*, for example, Cohen et al. (2007) describe hepatitis C as a 'shadow epidemic', as:

> One of the most clandestine of viruses...[It] infects healthy people who have no idea they are being attacked by something they can't even detect.

In all of these accounts the hepatitis C virus is constituted as resilient, cunning and sturdy. It can stay alive for up to four weeks, break skin, cross bodily boundaries, enter into bloodstreams, and through its own initiative 'leave the body of a person'. Hepatitis C might also 'creep' up unsuspectingly, a process presumably associated with its apparently 'slow moving' nature. It is 'clandestine' and difficult to detect. Reference to the human 'host' in the example above could be read in several ways, but the discourse clearly positions the host and the virus as adversaries. Here the 'host' is placid and inert, while the virus figures as insidious and calculating, as

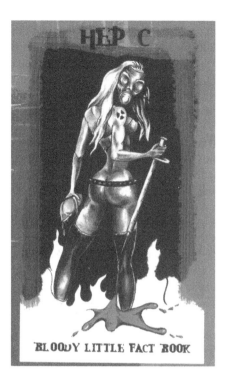

Figure 2.1   'Bloody Little Fact Book': Hepatitis C in health promotion

Source: The 'Bloody Little Fact Book' (Courtesy of Hepatitis Queensland, artwork by Rachel Otto).

always already seeking out environments most conducive to its survival. The sense we have is one of the virus laying in wait, circling, always already in preparatory mode, waiting to attack.

To a large extent, these renderings of the virus – as ubiquitous and sturdy – resonate with other research into how people interpret and imagine the virus (Davis and Rhodes 2004). Why might this overarching narrative and symbolic rendering of the hepatitis C virus have purchase? Within the present context, we argue that the rhetorical power of the single narrative lies in its close association with and reiteration of a set of broader understandings about people who inject drugs. Here, as we note in Chapter 3, there is a morphological connection between the meta-narrative of hepatitis C – which accounts for the virus as simultaneously hidden, sneaky, duplicitous, cunning, inconveniently persistent and unpredictable – and broader conceptualisations of people who inject drugs as similarly cunning, duplicitous, sneaky and unpredictable. As we know, hepatitis C and injecting drug use tend to be conflated (Harris 2005). The single narrative gains purchase from this conflation and the ongoing legacy of hepatitis C's symbolic adjacency to both injecting drug use and people who inject drugs. But the single narrative also obscures the purchase it gains from this conflation; in this sense we can say that through the single narrative 'what is ceaselessly perfected is a history of erasure' (Appelbaum 1995: 17). This is achieved primarily through the use of language of the kind we have just described, but also through visual renderings of hepatitis C. Much of the health promotion materials include imagery of the virus, injecting equipment, treatment, health care professionals and more. Speaking principally about art, Gordon Fyfe and John Law (1988: 2) have argued that visual depictions of a 'thing' function to simultaneously represent and constitute the thing itself, so that 'depiction, picturing and seeing are ubiquitous features of the process by which most human beings come to know the world as it really *is* for them'. Let us begin with an example of how this works, by considering an image that graces the cover of a small booklet about hepatitis C called the 'Bloody Little Fact Book' (Queensland Injectors Health Network 2007). This book is produced, importantly, for a specific audience: 'people' who inject drugs. Accordingly our interpretation of the booklet must be read with this target audience in mind.

This is an extraordinarily complex image of the virus, its subjects, objects and effects. How might we begin to unpack what is happening here? Let us start with the woman, who holds a liver in her left hand and a bloodied syringe in her right. She stands between health and illness: between the liver as a vital organ and source of health, to her left, and a needle, as source of danger, to her right. She might be a protector, a source of danger, or both. As we read it, her defiant and imposing stance, obvious physicality, prominent arm tattoo (bearing the symbol for radiation, and thus signalling toxins, poison or danger), firm grasp of the liver, and nuclear mask all point to her as a potent source of danger, threat or risk or as the embodiment of that danger, source or risk. It is also a sexualised depiction, one that suggests that the implicit target audience is heterosexual men. The particular configuration of subjects and objects, and the arrangement of the image, constitutes the female figure as a metaphor for the hepatitis C virus (which is constituted as danger, threat or risk). It also produces her as a metaphor for injecting drug use, so that injecting drug use is, in turn, produced and reproduced as a source of danger, threat or risk. When we suggest that she serves as a metaphor for both the hepatitis C virus and for injecting drug use, we are using a particular conceptualisation of metaphor that derives from the work of Ricoeur (1977), Derrida (1978) and others (Fraser and valentine 2008) and which claims that the literal and the metaphorical cannot be separated. In this sense, we are not arguing here that the metaphor of the dangerous subject simply references an *a priori* set of understandings of injecting drug use and people who inject drugs. Rather, it serves to constitute injecting drug use and people who inject drugs in particular ways: namely, as source of danger, threat and risk.

To this point we have said little about how gender figures in this image. Most obviously, to the extent that the female subject in the image figures as a metaphor for injecting drug use, danger, and risk, we can say that the image also constitutes femininity as source of danger and risk. Interestingly, this is not the only image

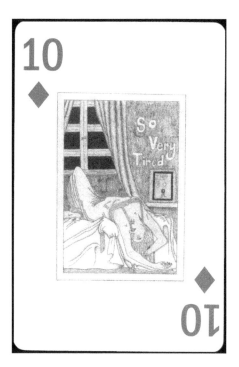

Figure 2.2   So very tired: Hepatitis C in health promotion

Source: From health promotion materials – a health promotion deck of cards distributed to prisoners and other individuals affected by HIV/AIDS and hepatitis C.

in the hepatitis C health promotion literature to feature so prominent a connection between woman and virus. The following image, for instance, is taken from a deck of cards produced by and for prisoners. The deck of cards is designed to raise awareness of blood-borne viruses and methods of prevention. We might again presume that the target audience is men. In this image, the woman lies draped across her bed, her back arched and chest pushed out, her breasts barely covered by her long, flowing dress. Her legs appear to be spread, her arms drag gently across the ground, her eyes are closed and her mouth is slightly open. Above her are the words 'So very tired', along with the phrase 'hep C+'.

On the one hand, the image is of a prone – possibly intoxicated – woman who appears weak, (sexually) vulnerable and fragile. As in the previous example, this is a sexualised depiction. The woman figures as an object of desire and as sexually passive. Both images render hepatitis C symbolically adjacent to, and the equivalent of, femininity. This is achieved through the depiction of the female subject as an object of temptation and desire, as seductive, a sexually alluring source of danger, and as constituted by irrationality and chaos. These are all features traditionally associated with the feminine (Fraser 2008). In this way,

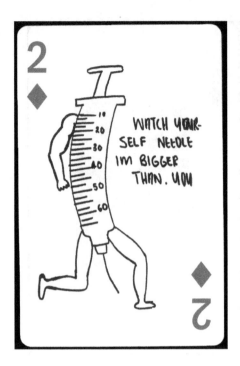

Figure 2.3   Watch yourself!: Hepatitis C in health promotion

Source: From health promotion materials – a health promotion deck of cards distributed to prisoners and other individuals affected by HIV/AIDS and hepatitis C.

hepatitis C figures not only as injecting drug use and as people who inject drugs, but also as femininity. Insofar as femininity is symbolically devalued, it becomes possible to say that hepatitis C health promotion materials produce an account of hepatitis C as virus/disease, injecting drug use and people who inject drugs as devalued. This has a range of potential political, ethical and material implications to which we shall return towards the end of this chapter.

Graphic renderings of hepatitis C as woman can be contrasted to other images appearing in the health promotion materials that equate health, vitality and purity with the masculine. In the same deck of cards, for example, the following image in Figure 2.3 appears.

The central image is of a needle with muscular arms and legs. Through a phallic metonymy, the image draws connections between injecting drug use (rendered through the needle) and masculinity (rendered through the muscular figure) and we read these connections in at least two ways. If we look more closely at the accompanying text, which reads 'Watch yourself needle I'm bigger than you', we see that the muscularity and size of the subject figures as a threat to the viability of the needle, which, as our preceding analysis demonstrates, appears as metaphor for danger/risk, and in turn as metaphors for hepatitis C, injecting drug use, people who inject drugs and femininity. So this image further constitutes the opposition between drugs/virus and 'host' as an extension of the binary logic which posits femininity and masculinity as symbolic opposites. Moreover, it operates to valorise masculinity at the same time as it operates to further devalue that which is symbolically associated with or adjacent to the feminine.

Bringing these threads of analysis together, then, we can identify a convergence between the virus, injecting drug use, people who inject drugs and addiction that renders the virus as:

– injecting drug use;
– people who inject drugs;
– addiction;
– femininity.

It also renders people who inject drugs as:

– the virus;
– injecting drug use;
– addiction;
– femininity.

And it also renders hepatitis C as:

– people who inject drugs;
– injecting drug use;
– addiction;
– femininity.

We now begin to have a sense of how the multiplicity of hepatitis C hangs together to produce a singular account of the virus/disease. The ontology of hepatitis C is achieved through the iteration, of gender symbolism and its symbolic, literal and material connections to injecting drug use and people who inject drugs. This singularity is achieved in one final way, and that is through its renderings of a key object alongside these enactments in hepatitis C discourses – the apparent target of the virus: the liver.

Prometheus' Liver

According to Greek mythology, Prometheus stole fire from Zeus and gave it to humans. Incensed, Zeus saw fit to punish Prometheus for the theft by abandoning him to the elements, tying him to a rock and leaving him to be attacked by animals. Each day an eagle visited Prometheus, pecking at his liver, and each night his liver regenerated. According to Power and Rasko (2008), there is considerable dispute in the literature about the meaning of Prometheus' crime and his punishment. One common view has been that his theft of fire 'was a crime of passion and his punishment targeted the bodily source of his impulsive behaviour' (Power and Rasko 2008: 425). A slightly different but related interpretation of ancient understandings of the liver is articulated by Hunt and de Luna (2007) who explain:

> In the ancient world, the liver was often understood as the seat of action that was sometimes called the 'heart' (as opposed to the mind) and very important in behavior [sic] and being as manifest by character.

In Hebrew, the word for liver is 'kabed', which in turn means 'weighty' or gravity'. The double meaning of this, according to Hunt and de Luna (2007) is the physical weight or size of the liver and the dignity or importance of the person. It is for these reasons that seers would engage in the practice of 'liver reading' in ancient times. Understood as the source of knowledge, wisdom and action, the liver was, for some, our most vital and fascinating organ. In these accounts we have a set of seemingly interrelated but somewhat incongruent interpretations of the symbolic meaning of the liver: as a source of action, as well as wisdom, as well as impulse. In our view, it is not necessary to draw any conclusions about which is the 'best' or most accurate interpretation of the liver's symbolic meaning. Instead, we are interested in how interpretations such as these might be brought to bear on our understandings of the liver and those diseases of the liver, of which hepatitis C is one.

In hepatitis C health promotion materials, the liver is frequently rendered as pure, virtuous, functional, orderly, heroic and – by extension – masculine. For example, one document (*Transmission Magazine*, 21 June 2009) describes the liver as an 'important' organ that 'always tries to repair itself after damage from things like drugs and alcohol and bad diet'. The 'special' qualities of the liver are regularly asserted in these materials: a unique organ with healing capacities and highly unusual attributes. The agency of the liver is regularly asserted, as in the above account, where the liver's capacity to 'repair itself' is detailed. Through these accounts, the liver comes to signify action, purity, performance, functionality and cleanliness. It is symbolically rendered in some accounts of hepatitis C as an organ of unique qualities and functions, and thus admirable, heroic and virtuous. How do these sketchings of the liver contribute to our understanding of 'what hepatitis C *is*'? They must be read alongside depictions of the virus as injecting drug use as source of threat and danger. This demands further consideration of the implications of the metaphorical chain of hepatitis C/injecting drug use/people who inject drugs/femininity as threat, danger and risk. Our question here is: a threat to what? If it is to the liver (one of the virus's principal targets) then it is also a threat to that which the liver symbolises. In particular, to the extent that the hepatitis C virus is constituted as a threat to the liver and all that it symbolises (purity, virtuosity, functionality, order, heroism and the masculine), anxieties surrounding the 'battle' between the virus and the liver reflect and reproduce a set of anxieties about the symbolic threat that femininity and drug use pose to the masculine order, and to freedom, enterprise, and rationality. Moreover, as the liver symbolises agency, action and freedom, hepatitis C/drug use emerges as symbol of drug 'addiction'. As Seddon (2007) and others (Fraser and valentine 2008; Lenson 1995) have pointed out, the origins of the word *addiction* are in the notion of attenuated free will, being derived from the relationship between slaves and their masters in Roman law. 'Addiction' is thus a commentary on free will and rationality, to the extent that the will of the 'addict' is understood as being attenuated, 'impaired' or 'violated' in some way (West 2001: 3). Because late modernity is characterised by a valorisation of agency, rationality, autonomy and choice, the diseased 'addict' is a symbol of horror because s/he signifies disorder, chaos, lack of control, uncertainty and irrationality (Seear and Fraser 2010). This, then, is the final observation we make about the 'holding together' of hepatitis C as singular. It is achieved through an enactment of a set of concerns about addiction, femininity, drug use and those who inject drugs, and the symbolic threat that they separately and collectively pose to freedom, rationality, enterprise and the masculine. As Mol reminds us, however, the point is not that hepatitis C *represents* these things. Rather, hepatitis C *is* all of these things (and others that we have not covered here). Its ontology is politics.

Conclusion

Science, Nelly Oudshoorn argues, has the 'capacity to create new things and new worlds' (Oudshoorn 1994: 43). Here, the materialisation of new 'things' and 'worlds' must be read as a product of its relation in space and time to health promotion – its specific purposes, actions, culture, presents, pasts and futures. Some of these were considered at the start of this chapter; it will be recalled, for example, that in practical terms, health promotion has emphasised self-care and care for others, instantiated via an ethic of individual responsibility for health, the precautionary principle, preventative action, and the importance of 'healthy living' (Bunton, Nettleton and Burrows 1995: 1). As Robin Bunton (1992: 9) has argued, 'populations [have become] subject to increasingly more pervasive methods' of health promotion, as virtually every aspect of existence becomes the object and subject of medical advice. Numerous commentators, adopting a broadly Foucauldian perspective, have been critical of health promotion policies and practices for this reason (Petersen and Lupton 1996; Bunton et al. 1995; Nettleton 1995, 1996; Bunton 1992; Lupton 1995; Petersen 1997a; Petersen 1997b; Castel 1991; Bunton and Burrows 1995; Daykin and Naidoo 1995). In political terms, health promotion functions to produce individual actions as the object of scrutiny and surveillance, linked, inextricably and forever more, to broader public health aims.

In this chapter our concern has been less with these individualising and responsibilising tendencies and aims of health promotion (as these have already been well documented elsewhere), including in our own work (Fraser 2004; Seear 2009a). There is no doubt that health promotion materialises responsibilised subjects through conduct and the 'conduct of conduct' (Foucault 1994). Doubtless, it is individualising in its effects. This much is implied in the Aristotle quote that opened this chapter:

> We are what we repeatedly do. Excellence, then is not an act, but a habit.
> (Aristotle, quoted in a safer injecting brochure detailing ways to prevent transmission of hepatitis C)

Health promotion demands 'excellence' in the sense of enterprise, individuality, autonomy and responsible action. Health promotion enacts its subjects as such, through processes of iteration. But the responsibilising and individualising tendencies of health promotion are not all that can be said. We need also to consider the *how* and *why* of health promotion, the ways in which health promotion materials handle, produce and materialise hepatitis C as an object, in spite of its contradictions, tensions, fragmentation and fissures. It concerns the reasons why these specific materialisations are necessary. As we noted at the outset, insofar as health promotion and the 'new public health' are to be understood as responsibilising in both intention and effect, disease demands to be produced as stable, coherent and singular, in spite of the multiplicity we have identified throughout this chapter. This is because certainty is productive to the extent that it permits injunctions to be directed towards subjects in which they must act upon themselves (and others). But, importantly, uncertainty is not entirely eschewed in health promotion. Uncertainty about symptoms, for instance, has its own unique and productive place in health promotion. It allows for an account of the hepatitis C virus as cunning, duplicitous and sneaky. Here uncertainty and variability figure as evidence not of multiplicity itself but – paradoxically – of singularity. It is, remarkably, the very proof of that which it simultaneously works to erase. This uncertainty, this multiplicity should produce questions about the stability and coherence of hepatitis C as material object. Crucially, and somewhat ironically, however, it actually serves as the 'glue' that holds the disease together. In turn it impacts on its subjects in new ways, demanding they improve their habits, be more attentive, stay on guard. It demands, to again quote Aristotle, nothing short of 'excellence'.

As we found in Chapter 1 when we examined medical literature, health promotion materials, educational efforts and harm reduction strategies reproduce understandings of how the virus 'works', 'moves', 'functions' and 'operates' that have the potential to shape both the subjects of the epidemic and its materiality. Most obviously, claims that hepatitis C is unpredictable, changeable, duplicitous, inconveniently persistent, sturdy and ubiquitous have ramifications for how we understand our capacity to prevent transmission. If the virus can 'sneak' or 'creep' up on its subjects, move around undetected, slip in and out of bodies seamlessly, break barriers and change its formation, then how are we to ever manage it? At one level the perception might be that hepatitis C is impossibly complex and unpredictable such that it is also ultimately unmanageable. We need to think carefully about how these renderings of the virus circulate through health promotion and educational efforts. To what extent, for example, do health promotion and harm reduction strategies assume *a priori* understandings of the virus as unmanageable and, in so doing, reiterate them, through, for instance, limiting suggestions about what can be done to avoid exposure to the virus? Where this occurs there are material consequences for the spread of the virus across populations and for the individuals so affected. With all of this in mind, we ask what alternative framings, if any, are available? As a starting point, we suggest moving away from accounts of the virus as duplicitous, unpredictable and cunning. Why do we not, instead, produce accounts of the extent to which medical knowledge and practice about the virus is partial, fragmented and limited? Why not account for variations in symptomatology as less a function of the virus' unpredictability and more a reflection of medicine's limited capacities to grapple with these variations? In rethinking how multiplicity is both depicted and 'refracted', we can render these limitations visible. The erasure of that which is too difficult or which does not fit is politically, ethically materially and personally productive. As Mol and Law remind us, indeed, much is at stake. But it might still be otherwise.

Chapter 3

Materialising Hepatitis C and Injecting Drug Use in Self-help Literature and Beyond

In the Introduction we noted that 'new consensus about illness is usually reached as a result of negotiations among the different parties with a stake in the outcome' (Aronowitz 1998: 1). This process of negotiation is mainly social, entailing a range of agents and a variety of discursive avenues. This is especially true for the blood-borne virus hepatitis C, the medical, social and political features of which – associations with injecting drug use, 'tainted blood' scandals and HIV – render it a controversial disease involving a range of highly motivated stakeholders. In this chapter we build on the analyses conducted in Chapters 1 and 2 by examining a third set of agents in the process Aronowitz identifies: self-help books on hepatitis C. In conducting this analysis we offer insights into two different but inevitably related areas: first, the content of the books and the way they construct hepatitis C and those who have it, and second, the ways in which the multiplicity and complexity of these constructions can best be understood so as to grasp effectively the social and political implications of disease. We ask a question that is both empirical and epistemological – a question at the core of this book: how might the complexities of the negotiations and meaning-making around hepatitis C be made sense of? This chapter aims to map three key issues helping to shape the way hepatitis C and those who have it are constituted in these books: HIV, injecting drug use and iatrogenic (medically caused) transmission.

The chapter is divided into two parts. First it will address its key question head on: how best to conceptualise the complexities by which hepatitis C is being constituted. Jacalyn Duffin's work on hepatitis C disease concepts will be revisited briefly. This will open out space to understand diseases in their complexity: as socially and politically located articulations of illness, rather than as stable, biologically self-evident phenomena beyond culture, history and politics. To enhance this discussion the work of John Law and Annemarie Mol will also be considered. This body of work pays close attention to the place of research in the constitution of realities. It asks probing questions about the processes of writing and about the importance of thinking through the political effects of research and writing. In asking how scholars might go about attempting to render phenomena such as diseases in all their complexity, it offers valuable insights for the analysis to be conducted here. Following this discussion the second section will examine a selection of self-help books written about hepatitis C since its naming in 1989. This exploration will allow us to spell out some of the key forces at work in the making of hepatitis C as it is understood today, and the ways in which these are framed and linked.

Approach: More than one and less than many

Thinking and writing the actions, associations and implications of a disease is no easy task. As with have noted, perhaps all, phenomena, diseases are almost literally unspeakably complex. At every stage of the process of articulation – that is, the thinking, speaking and writing – of disease, decisions about inclusion and exclusion, connection and separation, emphasis and de-emphasis are required. As we have noted, simplifications must be made so that the processes of articulation can be completed effectively or, at least, come to some kind of meaningful temporary halt. This is no less the case for hepatitis C than for other diseases; indeed, hepatitis C's highly politically charged associations mean that processes of articulation and choice register as especially significant in the thinking and writing. In managing this significance, we have turned to theorisations of complexity in the social sciences. How best to do justice to the complexity of hepatitis C, to engage its associations with equally complex phenomena such as HIV, injecting drug use and iatrogenesis in ways that render its specificities productively while enacting enough closure to allow meaning making?

Throughout this book we have argued that hepatitis C can be seen not as some kind of organic 'potsherd' (Duffin 2005) to be dug up and described by medical researchers. Instead, it is a continually iterated object – the description, metaphorical representation and treatment of which materially shapes it over time. As such, articulating it is complex and challenging. This book is an attempt to articulate this complexity, to 'walk' some of the multiple ways hepatitis C is iterated in cultural and social practices. Despite the breadth of our approach, we acknowledge that this undertaking can only ever be partial. This acknowledgment is not simply an exercise in conceding our limits. It also underpins a fundamental conceptual commitment of this book. Following the work of Mol and Law, we argue that simplicity and complexity should not be understood as polar opposites. According to Mol and Law (2002: 7) it is possible to identify 'a variety of orders – modes of ordering, logics, frames, styles, repertoires, discourses' operating in relation to any phenomenon. We do not live within a single episteme, they argue. Rather, we live simultaneously within multiple epistemes, multiple worlds that 'overlap and coexist' (2002: 8). For Mol and Law, 'multiplicity is thus about co-existence at a single moment' (2002: 8).

As Mol and Law point out, 'different modes of ordering or different styles of justification or different discourses may also overlap and interfere with one another' (2002: 10). Thus, different ways of thinking, speaking and doing hepatitis C do not exist in isolation from each other. Indeed the points at which they abut, at which simplifications encounter each other in moments of complexity, produce some of the most productive features of the phenomenon. Here, in order to grasp both the multiplicity and the singularity of hepatitis C effectively, we mobilise tools for analysing these ways of thinking, speaking and doing together. As Mol and Law put it, '[a]ttending to multiplicity, then, brings with it the need for new conceptualisations of what it might be to hold together' (2002: 10). Here is the key conceptual task for this chapter, one that builds on the analyses conducted in Chapters 1 and 2: identifying the ways in which multiple accounts of hepatitis C in the self-help books examined are held together to constitute the disease, and offering critical insights into them – that is, exposing where the work of 'holding together' must take place, and considering where different ways of holding and different combinations might produce hepatitis C, its implications and those affected by it, differently.

Making sense of hepatitis C through self-help

There is a growing literature examining the role and function of self-help literature for citizens of modern liberal democratic societies. To date, this literature has tended to focus on the ways the assumptions at work in self-help construct the reader, and the proper subject more broadly (see for example Rimke 2000; Hazleden 2003, 2009; Cherry 2008). This focus leaves many other effects of the self-help genre open to analysis. Just as self-help constitutes readers as subjects, it also constitutes the other phenomena it discusses. For example, as the second author of this book (Kate Seear) (2009a) notes, self-help material on endometriosis constitutes 'risk' and related ideas such as control and certainty. In the case of hepatitis C self-help literature, the phenomena constituted are many: the notion of disease, the disease hepatitis C itself, HIV, blood, infection, medicine, doctors, body parts such as livers, and so on. The particular character of these constructions is in many ways in keeping with broader ways of understanding the phenomena. Self-help articulates with broader discourses, after all. We will see, for example, links between assumptions made here and those made in the medical and health promotion literature already discussed. At the same time, self-help is also a literary genre. As such, it has its own conventions and demands. These conventions and demands uniquely shape the phenomena under discussion, and in doing so, exert pressure reciprocally on those ways of understanding operating in broader discourse. All these forces need to be taken into account when self-help material is analysed from the point of view of particular health problems or particular populations.

As Krug (1995) has noted self-help books form an important resource through which individuals make sense of hepatitis C. There are a surprisingly large number of such books, some aimed at those whose hepatitis C was medically acquired, some at 'recovered' injecting drug users, and others at anyone with the disease. Some are overtly medically oriented, others have a new age flavour, and still others rely on mainstream religious concepts. These variations shape the ways hepatitis C and those who have it are framed differently, yet there is some terrain all approaches tend to traverse. This chapter looks particularly closely at the constitution in self-help of two key issues for hepatitis C: 1. its links with HIV and; 2. an issue introduced in the previous chapter, agency and the divide between injecting drug use and iatrogenesis. In doing so, it identifies the constitution of a range of apparently collateral concepts and objects, examining how these turn out to bear on broader definitions of hepatitis C, its effects and those living with the disease. Questions of genre will be directly addressed. How do the norms of the self-help register bear on the ways the problem of hepatitis C is framed? As we will see, the emphasis in much of the material is on individual agency and self-efficacy as well as on questions of personal guilt, responsibility and anger. These tendencies help shape the way hepatitis C is discussed, the conceptualisation of disease and its meaning, and the place accorded to individual practice in creating change.

1. HIV and 'other such viruses'

The production of hepatitis C is profoundly intertwined with that of HIV. Partly because they are both transmitted via the blood, hepatitis C and HIV are often mentioned together, such as in hepatitis C prevention literature (Fraser and Treloar 2006). The histories of the identification and response to the two diseases are also profoundly linked (Duffin 2005). Given that incidence and prevalence, degree of infectiousness, effects and prognosis vary significantly between hepatitis C and HIV, however, this tendency to link the two diseases can be misleading as it creates the impression they share other characteristics such as rates of fatality among unmedicated patients (Harris 2005; Rhodes and Treloar 2008). Outside prevention and medical circles, hepatitis C is only rarely discussed openly (Harris 2005). When it is, according to Krug (1997) it is characterised by an absence of, or gaps in, meaning. In this way, at least, hepatitis C is treated rather differently from HIV, which has a far stronger public profile and is regularly discussed publicly. Between these two points – the tendency to treat HIV and hepatitis C as the same, and the tendency to treat them differently – are the specific social, cultural and technical practices and discourses that constitute hepatitis C.

The self-help literature on hepatitis C exhibits many of the same characteristics as the broader discourse around the disease. Hepatitis C and HIV are regularly mentioned together, and their effects compared.[1] In some cases, the tendency to confuse the two viruses is acknowledged directly. For example, in all editions of

---

1   Aside from the cases examined here, other examples include Dolan 1999: 52: '[Hepatitis C] is known to be able to survive in dried blood for longer periods than many other such viruses like HIV', and Washington 2000; xv: 'The headlines may have already told you that Americans, still reeling from AIDS, are just beginning to realise that we are sitting on an even greater viral time bomb – hepatitis C'.

one guide (Everson and Weinberg 1998, 1999, 2002, 2006: 8), one man living with hepatitis C ('Bob') is quoted as describing disclosure in the following way:

> Most of what [people] know about viruses has to do with AIDS, so you get a lot of weird stares and silences.

Here Bob is intimating that disclosing his hepatitis C status prompts unspoken speculation about his sexuality. The book does not record any more of Bob's comments on this. Considered from the point of view of Mol and Law's ontology, we are left to wonder how and to what extent the iteration of hepatitis C in such instances of disclosure reconstitutes the disease differently in the minds and material practices of those told. Is the meaning of the disease remade as a result of their conceptions of Bob and his sexuality, or rather, is it Bob who is remade in light of their assumptions about the disease? No doubt both the disease and those living with the disease are shaped by the act of disclosure. Equally, the iteration of such scenes of disclosure are acts of constitution themselves, shifting readers' understandings of hepatitis C and the stakes involved in acknowledging a connection with the disease. As the first author (Suzanne Fraser) has argued elsewhere in relation to methadone maintenance treatment (Fraser and valentine 2008), despite tendencies to see iteration (and its companion concept, repetition) as the antithesis of change, it is possible to argue that in its replaying and re-staging of actions and situations, iteration always entails the possibility of change. Importantly however, in that all four editions of the book include the same quotation, it seems the authors identify no change at all across a decade in how the two diseases are understood.

In other self-help books, HIV and hepatitis C are discussed together for quite different reasons. Another guide (Paul 2005: 244) states that:

> Because HIV is spread through blood and body fluids, and hepatitis C is spread through blood, many folks have both viruses.

This is quite a complicated statement that, despite its apparent self-evidence, carries several untenable assumptions. An important difference in the constitution of hepatitis C in different parts of the world such as the United States and Australia is the rate of co-infection with HIV. While HIV and hepatitis C are indeed both transmitted via blood-to-blood contact, the two viruses are not equally robust and infectious. Australia's early and effective public health response to HIV resulted in extremely low rates of transmission in that country, even among people who inject drugs. The same cannot be said for the US, where public health responses were slower and less innovative. Rates of transmission of HIV in this group are consequently much higher. Thus, while Paul's statement applies in one place, it does not apply everywhere.

Beyond questioning the general relevance of this statement – or, as Law might put it (2004), its 'portability' – we can consider its other implications. Significantly, it treats the rate of coinfection as a necessary effect of the disease's intrinsic attributes (its means of transmission). As the differences between the US and Australia indicate, however, effects of this kind cannot be taken for granted. Political and social variations can shape rates of transmission profoundly. This is a further sense in which Mol and Law's notion of multiplicity can be mobilised in relation to hepatitis C. The two political contexts can be seen as producing hepatitis C in two quite different forms. One is readily collapsed with HIV, and carries with it stigma (itself uniquely shaped by its geographical context) associated with HIV, while the other is quite distinct from HIV and carries quite different forms of stigma. Further, it is worth noting that the physiological effects and implications of HIV and hepatitis C differ depending on whether they occur in the body separately or together. That is, symptoms, disease progression and response to treatment all vary depending on whether the two diseases co-occur or not. These variations, too, can be said to create different diseases.

Of course, Paul's (2005) statement represents a widespread, commonsense approach to the meaning of disease. It sees diseases as self-evident, pre-existing entities awaiting discovery, their attributes stable and consistent across contexts. In his adoption of the colloquial expression 'folks', Paul is clearly aiming to avoid or diminish expressions of stigma: the text seeks to strike a friendly, non-judgmental note in referring to people with hepatitis C. Yet by treating the socially and politically produced effects of the disease as natural or inevitable – as the expression of the disease's intrinsic attributes – rather than as the product of social policy and the concepts, including stigmatising ones, informing this policy, it ignores the very political context in which the stigma it seeks to combat comes to be generated. This oversight is one our book seeks to challenge: disease must be denaturalised if its meanings and associations are ever to be made fully available to remaking. In the next section we will discuss a similar conceptual move which treats hepatitis C transmission as the inevitable outcome of the injection of illicit drugs. Here, our aim is to draw out how Law and Mol's questions about the options available for constituting material phenomena through social practice (including such avenues informed by social norms and assumptions as self-help literature) can be brought to bear on research into disease and how it is made. As has been noted, hepatitis C has been made in at least two different ways as a result of political and social differences: one, as a constant consort of HIV, and the other as overwhelmingly distinct from HIV. The health and social implications of these different productions of hepatitis C are entirely material in their form and impact, and it is this materiality that constitutes the political import of the ontological role of politics in the making of disease. If as Law and Mol say, there are alternatives ('options') available in the way material phenomena are constituted, and that we must ensure we are aware of the stakes involved in different formulations of materiality, then we are obliged to attend to the constitution of hepatitis C in these terms as well. The question remains, of course, how we might choose between alternatives. This, in our view, can never be resolved in principle; it must rather be negotiated socially as Aronowitz explains, but perhaps in a rather more sophisticated way than currently available to the parties involved.

Bruce and Montanarelli's (2007: xiii) self-help book also speaks of HIV and hepatitis C together. As above, their attributes are compared and contrasted:

> ... HCV is now being described as 'the new HIV'... Hepatitis C is much more common than HIV ... [It] is transmitted in similar ways to HIV, through blood exposures, from contaminated needles and occasionally from high risk sexual exposure. Like HIV, HCV is an RNA virus that changes over time ... Like HIV, there is no effective vaccine against HCV, nor is there likely to be one in the foreseeable future. Like HIV, HCV is common in underserved communities – the homeless, people in prison, minority populations, veterans.

The comparisons drawn here begin with observations about the nature of the virus and routes of transmission, and conclude with a comment about disadvantage. The use of the expression 'underserved' has a similar intent to that of the previous use of the expression 'folks'. It invites us to sympathise with those affected by hepatitis C. Interestingly, drug users are not included in this list of the underserved. Is this an intentional exclusion and if so, what might motivate it? Is there uncertainty about whether people who inject drugs have legitimate claims on services, or is there an awareness that to iterate the disease via the figure of the drug user is to narrow its meanings, heighten the 'stakes' around it, and overdetermine its material 'options', in undesirable ways? The implications of injecting drug use for attributions of responsibility, guilt and rights in relation to hepatitis C will be explored in detail in the next section. For now, the co-production of HIV and hepatitis C here is worth thinking through further. As is common in this material, the meanings and implications of hepatitis C are spelt out via the example of HIV. At first glance this might appear understandable, even natural. Are the two not, after all, akin? Comparing the hepatitis C self-help literature to the HIV self-help literature would be instructive here. Research on the HIV self-help literature is, unfortunately, scant. A brief look at relevant titles (Tacconelli 2009; Cichocki 2009; Tatchell 1997) makes clear, however, that no such reciprocal association is drawn between the two diseases in that literature. Clearly, the kinship of two diseases is contingent upon strategic and circumstantial factors. In short, it is an 'option'. Why do self-help discussions of hepatitis C depend so much upon references to HIV? A partial answer to this lies in the next issue to be considered: the relationship between injecting drug use and hepatitis C in the self-help literature.

2. Injecting drug use and iatrogenesis

At present the vast majority of new hepatitis C infections recorded in the developed world are attributed to injecting drug use. While the hepatitis C prevention education literature usually lists the many different ways hepatitis C is thought to be transmitted, including the sharing of tattoo needles and toothbrushes, most of this literature is nevertheless aimed at people who inject drugs. In this sense, as we have already noted, injecting drug use and transmission of hepatitis C are treated as one in the medical and health literature. In describing routes of transmission and recommending forms of behaviour, the prevention literature constitutes particular kinds of injecting subjects (Fraser 2004) and particular understandings of hepatitis C (Treloar and Fraser 2004; Fraser and Treloar 2006). These mobilise notions such as the responsible addict, and hepatitis C as pollution. Beyond the health promotion literature, the linking of hepatitis C to injecting drug use in more public contexts such as medicine and the media also acts to constitute affected individuals and the disease in particular ways. It is thought, for example, that hepatitis C's association with injecting drug use contributed to a slow policy response in that people who inject drugs were perceived to be disorganised, not easily reached, and unlikely to adopt prevention measures (Hulse 1997). As Hopwood and Southgate (2003) have argued, ideas about people who inject drugs have contributed to the spread of hepatitis C by shaping policy responses and prompting a judgemental approach among health professionals.

Yet, as we have already observed, hepatitis C also maintains historical associations with iatrogenesis. Prior to the introduction of blood screening (around 1990 in many countries), transfused blood and other blood products were a significant source of infection. In 2004, perceptions of an unnecessary delay on the part of the Red Cross in introducing screening led to the establishment of the Inquiry into Hepatitis C and Blood Supply in Australia. As in the US and Canada (Orsini 2002) there are concerns that this delay led to the unnecessary infections among transfusion recipients and other consumers of blood products, and this has prompted calls for compensation. These calls and the scrutiny under which modes of transmission have been placed mean affected individuals have come to be divided between the two categories identified in Chapter 2: blood product recipients as innocent victims of the disease (and, to some observers, of negligence) and people who inject drugs as guilty vectors of the disease. Duffin (2005) notes that the first group correspond with what is called within the philosophy of medicine the 'ontological' concept of disease, that is, a view that sees the cause of disease as external to the sufferer, such as a germ. The second group correspond with what is called the 'physiological' concept of disease, that is, a view that sees the cause of disease as originating within the sufferer, such as a gene or behaviour. Hepatitis C's alignment with both disease concepts in self-help, and the hierarchy this alignment produces/reflects, will be considered in detail in the analysis that follows. *Inter alia*, it is important to explore how these divisions impact on the constructions of self made available to readers.

The politics of assigning emotion

One of the most striking products of the association between hepatitis C and injecting drug use to be found in the self-help literature is the sometimes implicit, sometimes explicit, construction of guilt and shame around diagnosis.

A range of emotional responses (all negative) are canvassed in the literature. These include anger, helplessness, hopelessness and fear (Rhodes and Treloar 2008; Treloar and Rhodes 2009). As Everson and Weinberg (1998, 1999, 2002, 2006: 4) confidently assert:

> You're worried about yourself. You're worried about the people you love. You're angry. Perhaps you even feel ashamed.

Here, the key issue is the location of certain familiar emotions at the centre of the hepatitis C problem, and the need to resolve or manage these emotions if progress towards an acceptable outcome (be it emotional acceptance of the hepatitis C diagnosis, a higher quality of life with hepatitis C, or an actual cure) is to be made.

Most importantly in this context, the emotions cited are not always consistently assigned to individuals. Instead, a series of what emerge as normalising assumptions are sometimes made about the emotions individuals experience depending on the circumstances in which they contracted hepatitis C. In one of the most explicit examples of this, Bruce and Montanarelli (2007: 3) sympathise with their readers by speculating that:

> If you received contaminated blood products, you're most likely angry. Why did this happen to me? If you got hep C from sharing IV needles, you may have to deal with guilt. Why did I do this to myself? Your biggest challenge might be to forgive yourself.

In the section following this discussion we directly explore the constitution of agency and individual culpability ('Why did I do this to myself?') in the language the books use. Here, the focus is on the distribution of emotions and the political implications of this distribution. This quote makes what could be characterised as a commonsense observation. Iatrogenic infection produces anger. Injecting drug use infection produces guilt. There is no doubt that these responses do indeed occur in these neat arrangements for some individuals some times. Yet emotions are not so readily formed by assumptions. In one of the interviews conducted for the study on which this book is based[2], anger was the first emotion experienced by Ian (41), who had contracted the disease through sharing needles:

---

2   The interviews informing this book were conducted with individuals diagnosed with hepatitis C living in Melbourne, Australia (n=30). Interview participants were recruited with the aid of a range of services and organisations including Hepatitis C Victoria, Harm Reduction Victoria, and the primary health services Next Door and Health Works. Flyers advertising the study were supplied to these services, and an advertisement was also carried in Hepatitis C Victoria's magazine. Participants were offered a reimbursement payment of AUD$30 to cover their travel costs and time. The interviews were semi-structured in format. They were audio-recorded and transcribed verbatim then coded using the data

Ian: I read an article in the local paper about how hepatitis C was on the rise and was dangerous and that. And I realised I'd used needles and I shouldn't have, and I went to the doctor, I was worried that I contracted it, and I went to the doctor's and bingo, what do you know, it was positive, I had it.

Interviewer: Okay. So do you remember how you felt at the time?

Ian: Yeah, really angry at my friends who, myself, my friends and, [pause] mainly myself and my friends.

In this extract Ian explains that his diagnosis prompted strong feelings of anger, directed both at himself, and at others. He does not explain in detail the object of his anger, but the context suggests it relates to the needle sharing activity he participated in, and the role of his friends in passing on the infection to him. Here anger is personal, interpersonal and local.

Another of our interview participants, Stacey (24), also expresses anger on diagnosis, but hers is quite a different reaction from that described by Ian:

Interviewer: And what did the doctor tell you at the time about hep C do you remember? When you first got diagnosed?

Stacey: He told me and I stormed out, I didn't want to talk to him. I cracked the shits, I thought he was lying so I went to another doctor. He said the same thing and I stormed out. And then I went and spoke to my drug and alcohol counsellors, that's how I found out about it, like what it does, and I got the book and all that kind of crap about it. And yeah, I looked right into it.

Interviewer: Why did you crack the shits?

Stacey: Because I thought he was lying to me, to be honest with you. I'm like 'no, bullshit, I couldn't', I just thought it wasn't possible, from stepping on a syringe, get fucked, you know what I mean, that's what I thought. And I said that to him 'get fucked, there's no way'. And I walked down to another doctor, got a blood test and he said the same thing, I went 'all right, thanks' and walked out. I don't like doctors, I don't go to doctors. I've gone to a doctor twice since I've been pregnant, so I'm not a doctor person, I can't handle them. They tell you too much, they think they know you, but as far as I'm concerned you know your body better than anyone. So when you're telling them something and they're saying 'no, it's not that', it shits me, so I tend to walk out and not listen to them.

---

management program, NVivo. The codes were derived with reference to the existing literature on hepatitis C, theoretical concepts, and the aims of the study. This study has been approved by the Monash University Human Research Ethics Committee (approval no. CF08/0426 – 2008000183).

As in Ian's case, anger is not, of course, confined to those who acquired hepatitis C iatrogenically. Stacey had been injecting drugs from the age of 12. In her interview she describes injecting heroin with friends on a beach, and inadvertently stepping barefoot on a syringe in the sand. This is how she explains her infection, as she also states that she did not share injecting equipment with others. Stacey's anger is largely directed towards the medical profession whom she identifies as controlling and complacent. In this sense, her anger is unlike Ian's in that it is directed unequivocally outwards, and incorporates a broad structural critique of sorts in its challenge to medicine's power and influence.

Another participant in the study, Spike (41)[3], also expresses strong feelings of anger following his diagnosis in the early 1990s:

> I was angry at the world, I was angry at myself. I thought, if only – 'if only' (laughs) – but you see, we didn't know. And there was no access ... to clean needles and syringes.

Spike is lamenting his own lack of knowledge about hepatitis C here, but also notes two important structural constraints on his own ability to protect himself against infection. First, at the time of his infection hepatitis C had not yet been identified by medicine, and second, needle and syringe programs were not available at the time, so sharing injecting equipment was very difficult to avoid. Like Stacey, Spike does not blame himself alone, but the factors he points to, and the sources of his anger are quite different.

Clearly these responses do not fit conveniently into Bruce and Montanarelli's (2007) typology whereby those who acquired hepatitis C by medical means (and, the implication is, by no fault of their own) experience feelings of anger, while those who acquired it through drug use (and thus, it is suggested, by their own flawed actions) experience feelings of guilt. Instead, the latter group find much to be angry about, as well as much to regret in their own actions. Untidy as they are, these emotions do of course make sense. Indeed, they raise important issues for drug policy in that they point to the transmission of disease as a social and cultural process as much as an individual one. Where anger is allotted in the literature only to those infected iatrogenically, an implication is created that other instances of transmission are entirely the product of individual failings (thus the allocation of guilt in these cases). In other words, to erase the possibility that people who inject drugs might experience anger about their infection is to erase responsibility for the epidemic for anyone but those people themselves. This set of meanings, this process of iteration in discourse has, of course, a parallel in practice in that individual concepts of

---

3 Here the participant is speaking in an interview he gave for a radio program produced as part of the research project on which this work is based ('Getting Clear', ABC Radio National documentary produced by Suzanne Fraser, technical production by John Jacobs. Aired November 28, 2009. Details available at: http://www.abc.net.au/rn/360/stories/2009/2748617.htm).

agency shape the number, scale and character of prevention strategies put in place (Fraser 2004). These strategies, their limitations and the specific points at which, or conditions under which, they fail, in turn shape the hepatitis C epidemic and the context in which new infections might or might not occur. For example, where agency and responsibility are conceived individually, the packaging and provision of safe injecting equipment are also conceived individually (single syringes, water capsules, spoons and so on). In that injecting often occurs in groups and within couples, and indeed, the majority of new hepatitis C infections are thought to occur in couples (for Australian figures, see National Centre in HIV Epidemiology and Clinical Research 2008a), this individualising assumption represents at best a lost opportunity to supply people who inject drugs with equipment in ways meaningful to their injecting practice.

Agency and infecting the self

The distinction made between anger and guilt points to a broader issue in the material: that of the location of agency. Where iatrogenesis is assumed to be the product of negligent or even malign agency on the part of authorities and those institutions invested with trust and responsibility, guilt is assumed to be the product of negligent (and even malign or self-destructive) agency on the part of hepatitis C positive persons. The latter form of negative agency is communicated in some explicit statements, but also via a range of statements where individual agency in contracting hepatitis C is implied through relatively subtle grammatical strategies. These echo very closely those found in health promotion literature. Thus, for example, Everson and Weinberg (1998: 31; 1999: 32; 2002: 32; 2006: 30) explain that:

> Many drug addicts share needles. They spread hepatitis C among themselves and maintain a pool of affected people.

Here, agency is established by the use of active voice. 'Addicts' 'spread' hepatitis C 'among themselves' and 'maintain' a pool of affected people. The expression used here so explicitly constructs agency on the part of the drug users that it almost reads as though this spread and maintenance are intentional. In another example, Paul (2005: 169) states that:

> Even if you already have hepatitis C, you're endangering yourself by continuing to use drugs.

In this example, people who inject drugs are advised that continuing to consume drugs can accelerate the negative effects of hepatitis C. For the argument being made here, the phrase 'you're endangering yourself' is of most relevance. A more directly responsibilising assertion is difficult to imagine, despite widespread recognition that the harms implied are as much the product of social, political and legislative *context* of consumption as they are of the drugs themselves or the individuals involved (Keane 2002). Noteworthy is the fact that although hepatitis C health information continually nominates alcohol consumption as the single most harmful factor for those with the disease, discussion of it is far from equally responsibilising in this text. Instead, statements such as the following are used: 'Alcohol can damage the body...' (Paul 2005: 168). In this case, the use of the word 'can' moderates the assertion being made. More importantly, the negative agency is located, in this case, in the substance itself rather than in the individual consuming the substance. A statement equivalent in tone to the one made about illicit drugs earlier might, for example, read as, 'If you continue to drink, you endanger your health'.

In a more complicated case, Bruce and Montanarelli (2007: 3-4) attempt to reassure drug using readers by insisting,

> ...however you got this disease, you don't deserve it. Hep C is not a punishment, and at this point it isn't productive to dwell on what you could have done to avoid getting hep C.

They go on to expand on the last part of this statement later: 'Don't ask what you could have done differently. Ask what you can do now' (2007: 4). Here, the aim of the comments is to offer comfort, at the same time that two other factors are suggested. The first, most explicit, is that it is now time to become active in health management, and the second, rather less directly expressed, is that there were indeed actions and measures that the reader could have taken to avoid acquiring hepatitis C. This is, of course, not an inaccurate statement. Our point here is not that hepatitis C is completely impossible to avoid. Rather, it is that suggestions of individual agency and responsibility are not consistently made, and that their presence or absence has a political valency. Many scholars have by now noted the centrality of individual responsibilisation for health and well-being to contemporary public health strategies and measures (see Fraser 2004 for a summary of this literature). They have criticised this approach arguing that structural factors shape health as much as or more than individual factors, and that often structural support is not available to make individualising exhortations to health realistic or fair. Thus, current or past drug injectors are not alone in being constituted as responsible for their health and as having failed to maintain their own physical well-being. However there are important differences between the many responsibilised groups, and these render this argument more pressing for some than others. The illegal, stigmatised nature of opiate and amphetamine injection, the limited availability of sterile syringes (almost impossible to acquire in some places, even today) and the dilemmas attendant upon medical engagement generally, and testing and diagnosis in particular, mean that this group is even less suited to statements that take for granted that the acquisition of disease could have been readily avoided through individual self-management, and assert that such self-management is now the most salient priority.

The dynamics of agency and responsibility found here are of course partly a product of the literary genre being analysed. Self-help literature is, by definition, predicated on the possibility that individuals can act to improve their circumstances, and that this action on the self is the key determinant of well-being (Rimke 2000; Cherry 2008). Thus, the individualising and responsibilising cast of the material is not altogether attributable to perceptions of the groups being addressed. As noted above however, this cast is especially questionable in this field as those addressed by the literature have, by and large, less access to the material and cultural resources likely to enhance control of individual destiny and circumstances. As also already noted, the responsibilising cast is not consistently found in the literature. Some individuals, practices and phenomena are linked to individual responsibility more than others, and the patterns for this map quite neatly onto mainstream moral values, for instance, those relating to illicit drug use as compared with alcohol consumption. In this sense, while genre cannot be ignored in the interpretation of the concepts and values mobilised in the literature, neither can it be seen alone to account for them. Indeed the previous chapter demonstrated the presence of very similar discourses of agency and responsibility in a very different literature.

Risk and causation

Accompanying this uneven attribution of agency in the literature is an equally politically inflected tendency to confuse causation. The first example of this tends to conflate injecting with transmission, only, however, in the case of the injecting of illicit drugs. So Everson and Weinberg (1998: 33; 1999: 34; 2002: 34; 2006: 31) state that:

> If you shoot up once, you may or may not get hepatitis C. But if you shoot up many times, you can almost count on it. The best way to avoid the risk is to avoid illicit intravenous drugs and to teach the next generation to avoid this dangerous behaviour.

The causation chain implied in this statement is both inaccurate and vague. 'Shooting up' or injecting substances does not in itself cause hepatitis C. Only the presence of the hepatitis C virus in the equipment used to inject, or in the substance injected, can cause transmission. Given that countless injections occur in medical and domestic settings (as in the treatment of diabetes) every day where hepatitis C is not transmitted, the chain of causation suggested here is inaccurate in at least two ways: 1) the injection of *illicit* substances is assumed to eventually lead to infection, and; 2) the injection of licit substances is ignored, implying no risk of infection occurs in this context. It is conceivable that were attitudes less explicitly set against injecting drug use, the measures proposed to curb infection would be rather more specific and evenhanded. To draw a comparison, this recommendation is akin to arguing, as once was common, that gay men should give up sexual intercourse so as to avoid contracting HIV. Such a recommendation would now be labelled unreasonable and even homophobic in Western liberal democracies.

In a different example of this tendency to misrepresent causation, Paul (2005: 21) states that:

> Healthcare professionals who treat people with hep C shouldn't judge you for your past or current behaviour that may have caused your hep C.

Clearly, as with some examples analysed earlier, this statement is intended to support readers. Yet the implication that individual behaviour 'causes' hepatitis C hints at a less tolerant approach. The word 'cause' is used quite broadly here. Yes, there is no doubt that without injecting, hepatitis C would not have been transmitted. Equally, however, other phenomena were also necessary to transmission. The presence of the virus in the population of people who inject drugs at a sufficiently high level of prevalence is also necessary. This prevalence rate is the product of a range of factors including the delay in identifying the disease and in producing and implementing screening and testing for it, the multiple use of injecting equipment in past and present population-level vaccination programs around the world, and the stigma associated with illicit drug use leading to barriers in accessing sterile equipment. If causation can indeed be spoken of as broadly as is suggested by the quotation, then many other factors, most of which are beyond the control of affected individuals, can also be said to 'cause' hepatitis C. As with the erasure of the possibility of anger about infection among people who inject drugs, the erasure of alternative 'causes' of hepatitis C also implies purely individual culpability. Further, the contribution of these other forces shaping, even driving, the epidemic, are obscured, and the need to engage them or, to put it in Mol and Law's terms, to comprehend hepatitis C as ontologically constituted by social and political decisions and practices; as re-makeable – even now – via alternative iterations; as literally held together in current forms by norms, assumptions and practices, and as such to act differently, is overlooked. If disease is made in its materiality by convention, practice and discourse, all these must be investigated to enable change. At present hepatitis C is confronted using many of the selfsame stigmatising phenomena that materialise it, and continue to hold it together as it is, in the first place.

Conclusion: Iteration, complexity and multiplicity

It is this last point, finally, that makes the question of how hepatitis C is constituted in discourse so pressing. As we also saw in Chapters 1 and 2, responses to the disease, attempts to alleviate stigma and impact positively on individual health and well-being often iterate key phenomena in the very ways that produce the problems of stigma and blame themselves. Conventional notions of guilt and innocence are reiterated via subtle expressions of sympathy and support. Causation is differentially iterated depending on the substance consumed, and agency and emotion are deployed in uneven ways depending upon assumptions about individual and structural culpability. Comparisons with HIV erase the social and political processes that shape the character and impact of disease. None of these effects are desirable, yet it is important to recognise that they are also not exhaustive. As Law and Mol have argued, phenomena are constituted multiply, not as different aspects or perspectives, but as different objects in their materiality. We must not oversimplify the effects of multiple and paradoxical expressions such as those both sympathetic and foreclosing. Here we face epistemic complexity or contradiction: discourse that is at once, for example, committed to non-essentialising constructions (of the changeable, redeemable self) and essentialising constructions (of the bounded, predictable, identifiable disease). To reduce these complexities in purely negative assessments, or in bland assertions of plurality, would be to relinquish the very critical purchase an analysis of this kind must offer. Yet, as Law and Mol have also argued, denying the need to simplify is disingenuous and equally counterproductive. Where does this leave us in understanding the constitution of hepatitis C and those affected by it, and in formulating responses? In Law and Mol's terms, hepatitis C must be understood as more than one and less than many. This is undoubtedly an awkward ontological space to occupy. Here it helps to return to the key questions an ontological politics proposes:

1. Where are the options?
2. What is at stake?
3. Are there really options?
4. How should we choose?

Above we have examined some of the options in self-help for the materialisation of hepatitis C and related phenomena. We have considered the stakes in these materialisations, and now, given those stakes emerge as significant, there is a need to consider how to choose new, or more careful, or more responsive, iterations. Of course, these questions have a very specific concern. They ask not what options are available for representation, for the act of *reflecting* the materiality of prior phenomena in different ways, but for *constituting* phenomena in their materiality in different ways through iteration. Where hepatitis C is iterated as HIV's necessary consort or as inevitably arising from injecting, the measures taken to respond to the disease reify these attributes in practice. Automatic testing for hepatitis C among those with HIV, for example, is one way of shaping epidemiological knowledge on this issue (see Aronowitz 1998, for a discussion of this dynamic in other disease contexts). Associating hepatitis C with HIV, and inadvertently implying similarity between the two in relation to the poor prognosis attributed to untreated HIV risks contributing to the scale of the epidemic by prompting despondency and fatalism in some cases (Fraser and Treloar 2006). These are some of the ways hepatitis C, multiply produced in different contexts or according to different pieces of knowledge, can be understood as more than one and less than many – as materially distinct entities that are never entirely independent of one another. This multiplicity, operating in self-help, as well as in health promotion and medical literature, represents both the problem and the potential for generating change in hepatitis C epidemics.

Chapter 4

Knowing, Doing, Hoping: Diagnosis and the Limits of Biological Citizenship

'What can I know? What must I do? What may I hope?'

(Immanuel Kant, quoted in Rose 2007a: 257)

'... don't you have a relationship with yourself?'

(Giuseppe, male, 41 years)

As we have seen, health promotion and self-help literature consistently frame people with hepatitis C as responsible subjects in charge of managing their own health. People who inject drugs who have been diagnosed with hepatitis C must engage with these injunctions to health and self-care in unique ways. Their status as 'addicts' sees them medicalised as illegitimate risk takers suffering from a 'disease of the will' and thus lacking self-control. Their status as hepatitis C patients medicalises them in quite a different way: as potentially active and self-regulating health consumers necessarily open to taking legitimate corporeal risks, such as those courted in treatment. In this chapter we draw on in-depth, semi-structured interviews conducted with hepatitis C-positive people who inject drugs in Melbourne, Australia, to consider this tension. We do this by exploring the insights made available by the encounter between Nikolas Rose's theorisation of biological citizenship, and participants' responses to their hepatitis C diagnoses. What does it mean to be addressed as a choosing, responsible subject largely by virtue of potential exposure to, or acquisition of, a virus? What does it mean in the context of injecting drug use and the many challenges associated with it to be encouraged to undergo an onerous form of treatment, the outcome of which is highly uncertain, or to be told to make significant lifestyle changes, when no symptoms are present? How, in short, do people who inject drugs respond to the contrary and intensely morally inflected injunctions to biological citizenship thrown up by the collision of two key ideological notions in the West: addiction and infectious disease? What do their circumstances and responses tell us, in turn, about the nature and limits of contemporary forms of biological citizenship and for public health more broadly? This chapter addresses all these questions, concluding by considering a further question – one too infrequently explored in detail in this field – what have been the political effects of the medicalisation of addiction, and what are the limits of the strategy of medicalisation?

The analysis undertaken in this chapter was initially prompted by a key trend visible in our interviews with people diagnosed with hepatitis C.[1] These interviews

---

1   See pp. 73-4.

indicated that some people who inject drugs do not pursue information and advice about hepatitis C after diagnosis, and that the information initially accessed in the diagnostic clinical encounter sometimes forms the only knowledge acquired, and the only basis on which health and self-care decisions are made, for many years following diagnosis. In an important sense, these participants turned away from medicine almost as soon as their condition, and for some, their symptoms, had been medicalised (that is, framed in medical terms, considered constitutive of a disease, understood to be amenable to medical intervention). How should this turn be viewed? What is behind it, and how does it fit with contemporary public health pressures to engage 'health' and medicine continuously? This chapter extends the insights developed in previous chapters which highlighted the limits of medical approaches to disease, aiming to answer these questions first by placing addiction and hepatitis C diagnosis in context. Examining briefly contemporary approaches to the politics of medicalisation, we argue that the critique of medicalisation launched in the 1970s but still operating in a range of forms today functions at something of a tangent to the concerns of highly marginalised groups such as people who inject drugs. Yet as the interviews analysed here show, some of the critique's observations are especially relevant to hepatitis C. In the following section we turn to material on biological citizenship that in many ways forms an extension of these approaches in that it actively poses relations between individuals and biomedicine in new ways. We pay particular attention to the fit between these ideas and the unique status of people who inject drugs in Western liberal democracies. In the last substantive section we go on to consider these insights in direct relation to the accounts of engagement with medicine provided by the individuals interviewed for this book. The aim is not so much to 'test' biological citizenship theory against the case of injecting drug use and hepatitis C. Rather, it is to deploy this theory in a particularly challenging context to discovery what is thrown up by the tensions that emerge.

Background

To date, public health attempts to radically reduce rates of hepatitis C transmission have failed, although this does not mean reductions have not occurred. Reports of new infections in Australia, for example, fluctuated between 355 and 520 between 2003 and 2007 (National Centre in HIV Epidemiology and Clinical Research 2008b). While the hepatitis C prevention literature usually lists the many different ways the disease is thought to be transmitted (including via the sharing of tattoo needles and toothbrushes), as we have seen, most of this literature is aimed at people who inject drugs. In Chapter 2 we argued that, in describing routes of transmission and recommending forms of behaviour, the prevention literature constitutes particular kinds of injecting subjects (see also Fraser 2004) and particular understandings of hepatitis C (see also Treloar and Fraser 2004; Fraser and Treloar 2006). These mobilise notions such as the responsible addict, and hepatitis C as pollution. The linking of hepatitis C and injecting drug use in other contexts, such as the media and medical literature, also acts to constitute affected individuals and the disease. As we noted, (Hopwood and Southgate 2003), ideas about injecting drug users have contributed to the spread of hepatitis C by shaping policy responses and prompting a judgemental approach among health professionals. The prohibitionist legal background to injecting drug use is also central to this. All these ideas and assumptions have contributed to the materiality of the disease: its prevalence and population concentration.

Treatment for hepatitis C has also been shaped in part by ideas about affected individuals. For example, until relatively recently (2001), government-funded treatment for hepatitis C in Australia was not offered to people who inject drugs. It was thought that such patients would not be organised enough to complete the treatment program (Stoové et al. 2005). Implicit in this arrangement was the recognition that treatment for hepatitis C was onerous. This is still the case. Depending upon genotype, degree of liver damage, age and clinical markers, patients face either 24 or 48 weeks of treatment. During this time they can experience a range of debilitating side effects including fatigue, gastrointestinal disturbances, flu-like symptoms, major depression and anxiety (Hopwood and Treloar 2005; Fried 2002). Moreover, historically, cure rates have been very low. In recent years, the uncertainty surrounding the likelihood of cure has been reduced to some extent by new treatment regimes. Individuals with some genotypes of hepatitis C now have up to 80 per cent chance of cure. New research argues that treating early, even where symptoms are absent, increases the likelihood of cure. Under these conditions, where the chance of cure has risen but is by no means sure, and the treatment is long and taxing but increasingly promoted, uncertainty prevails.

As we have noted, being diagnosed with hepatitis C impacts on individuals in a range of ways. These can be divided into two main areas. Firstly, aspects of the politics of the disease – stigma and discrimination – shape affected individuals' sense of self, for example, through concern around disclosure (Harris 2005, Hopwood and Southgate 2003, Anti-Discrimination Board of NSW 2001) and reminders of a past, since disavowed, self (Hopwood and Southgate 2003). In addition, characterised by judgemental attitudes and poor levels of professional knowledge, interactions with general practitioners and other healthcare professionals can prompt shame and a sense of marginalisation (Fraser and Treloar 2006; Hopwood and Southgate 2003). As an important Australian inquiry found (the NSW Anti-Discrimination Board Inquiry into Hepatitis C-related Discrimination 2001), medical care is a main site of discrimination. Secondly, the ways in which hepatitis C is still 'under construction' medically impact on the meaning of a diagnosis and its effects on identity. Several factors – continuing uncertainty around symptoms on the part of health professionals even after diagnosis, related uncertainty surrounding the different degrees to which individuals experience symptoms, and the extended progression of the disease in which symptoms may or may not emerge over decades – mean that a medical diagnosis can instate uncertainty and confusion as much as clarity. Questions remain about what a hepatitis C diagnosis means for the body, and thus for the subject. How do all these uncertainties characterising hepatitis C contribute to the reshaping of identity? Most importantly for this chapter, how well does the main option available for revising identity – medicalising the self – serve affected individuals?

The critique of medicalisation

The role of medicine in daily life has long been the subject of intense critical attention. Emerging in the 1970s, critiques of what was framed as the medicalisation of Western liberal society have made major contributions to sociology, feminist studies, ethnography and other social sciences. Deborah Lupton (1997: 95) summarises the critique in the following way:

> Supporters of the medicalisation critique have generally identified a central paradox ... despite its alleged lack of effectiveness ... and iatrogenic side-effects [Western medicine] has increasingly amassed power and influence. They contend that social life and social problems have become more and more 'medicalised', or viewed through the prism of scientific medicine as 'diseases'.

For some, such as Zola (1972), this process of medicalisation has seen medicine increasingly act in a regulatory mode reminiscent of the action of religion and the law. In Illich's view (1975), it has been the basis for a decline rather than an improvement in health. What has been the function of this process of medicalisation? Some have argued explicitly that medicalisation is contemporary society's means of dealing with deviance. Conrad and Schneider (1980a) identified three main implications of the process. First, medicalisation tends to relieve 'deviants' of at least some of the moral responsibility for their behaviour. Second, within a medicalising framework, punitive responses become less common than therapeutic ones. Third, medicalisation allows the medical profession to garner increasing authority over the management of deviance.

More recent approaches to medicalisation have complicated the picture drawn during the 1970s, documenting the way in which health conditions move out of, as well as into, the purview of medicine depending upon changing social behaviour, and concepts of normality and health (Turner 1995, Porter 1997). According to Scott (2006: 134), who has written on the medicalisation of shyness, 'trends of both medicalisation and demedicalisation can be observed, although the former seems to be outpacing the latter'. Scott's observation reflects a major shift in approach to medicalisation since it was first elaborated. Many scholars now consider the earlier work to have overstated the power of medicine and underestimated the role patients play in both encouraging medicalisation and resisting it. Ballard and Elston argue (2005: 228), for example, that 'some earlier accounts of medicalisation over-emphasised the medical profession's imperialistic tendencies and often underplayed the benefits of medicine', assuming a docile populace at the mercy of medicine bent on expansion and control. In their view, the advent of the 'postmodern era' and the related de-centring of rationalism and science suggest the prospect of *decline* in the influence of medicine, and a decrease in medicalisation.

Other critics offer a range of different views while uniting in the conviction that the picture of medicalisation must be drawn more subtly than it was initially. Labelled a 'cliché' by Nikolas Rose (2007b: 700), the traditional medicalisation critique has given way to analyses that identify different aspects of medicalisation. Conrad and Schneider (1980b), for example, responded quickly to early criticisms of their work by naming three different levels of medicalisation: conceptual, institutional and interactional. Ballard and Elston (2005: 235) observe that elaborations such as these 'provided a framework within which it becomes possible to recognise that there might be different degrees of medicalisation; that the different dimensions of medicalisation might not always co-exist in close parallel; and that demedicalisation along one or more dimension might also occur'.

Another way of looking critically at the question of medicalisation beyond degrees and levels of medicalisation is of course via the question of power relations between patients and other elements that make up medical phenomena. As already noted, patient agency in relation to medicalisation was frequently neglected in early accounts. Bringing this factor into analyses recasts medicalisation both in terms of questions of force and regulation and in terms of the category of the medical itself. Patients are now recognised as intrinsic to medicine, rather than merely the 'targets' of it. The consumer health movement has played a significant role in extending patients' place and activity within medicine, though this is not to say patients were not active before. And while this change has brought many benefits, it has not done so without generating some problems too. Patients can no longer take refuge in the notion of medicine's benign paternalism. They must make their own decisions, and operate as rational consumers even while ill and under pressure. It is the individual patient's right (and responsibility) to make independent, informed decisions based on the facts as provided by medical practitioners, and to ensure they are not subject to undue influence by practitioners. As Nancy Tomes (2007: 698) puts it, 'In the new era of collaborative medicine, patients have nowhere to hide'. As do other scholars, however, Tomes makes clear that there can be no going back. Medicalisation as a general development cannot be reversed. Rose (2007b) goes further than this, making the point that, much more than something we might reject or turn back from to regain a prior state, contemporary medicine 'has made us what we are'. And what we are is complex and contradictory, as is the nature of medicalisation itself. In his view, we must make the idea of medicalisation the starting point for any analysis of the merits or otherwise of treatment or other health measures and innovations, rather than a diagnostic end point characterised by clichés and generalisations.

Medicalising addiction

This observation is especially relevant to this chapter in that hepatitis C and the great majority of individuals directly affected by it (people who inject drugs) pose unique questions for medicalisation. Over the last few decades both injecting drug use and hepatitis C have been intensively linked to medical frameworks, yet their social and cultural locations trouble straightforward statements about the effects of these linkages. The designation of the hepatitis C virus as separate from the hepatitis A and hepatitis B viruses is a relatively recent event (1989). Prior to this, as we have noted, hepatitis C was described only in terms of that which it was not, in that it was called 'non-A, non-B hepatitis'. With the identification of the virus came the development of treatment medications and screening processes, both for the purposes of diagnosis and for the testing of donated blood. While anecdotal reports and clinical experience had long suggested the existence of 'another hepatitis', it was the naming process that allowed the rather diverse and sometimes elusive range of bodily symptoms described by individuals to be codified as signs (Duffin 2005) and enfolded into medical processes and frameworks.

Perhaps paradoxically, the even more elusive condition of addiction has experienced a far longer history of medicalisation. It is worth looking briefly at this history because it bears directly on the central questions posed in this chapter: how should we understand the politics of medicalisation in relation to addiction? In turn, how should we view the opportunities and injunctions associated with medicalisation and contemporary biological citizenship as they relate to people who inject drugs affected by hepatitis C?

William White (1998, 2001) has written in detail on the rise of the disease model of addiction. He identifies a number of 18th and 19th century texts in which medical approaches to 'drunkenness' are developed, and argues that these would later become the 'building blocks of the modern disease concept of alcoholism'. The features of this approach to drunkenness were:

- Biological predisposition (heredity);
- Drug toxicity (or the effects of the substance itself);
- Morbid appetite (or craving);
- Pharmacological tolerance;
- Disease progression;
- Inability to refrain from consumption;
- Loss of volitional control over quantity of intake;
- Negative biological, psychological and social consequences of chronic consumption.

In the process of making this case for disease, the early writings struggle, White points out, to distinguish drunkenness as a vice from drunkenness as a disease. While there were a range of factors driving the development of the medicalisation of addiction, this was one of the strongest – the shared view that an approach to regular drug use was needed that exceeded the traditional view of it as a moral failing or a sign of wickedness. As Levine (1978) also argues, the desire to reduce the stigmatisation of regular drug users has been behind much contemporary enthusiasm for a medicalised approach.

White further notes that the disease concept of addiction translated readily in the 19th century from alcoholism to opiate use. Widely disseminated throughout society due to the prevalence of infectious disease and painful medical disorders at that time, opiates alleviated, as White puts it, 'what medicine could not cure' (2001: np). While in earlier centuries the idea that one could become addicted to opiates – dependent on them physically and likely to suffer from withdrawal symptoms if access was lost – was unknown, by the 19th century it was becoming widely accepted, largely in response to perceptions of opium use as destroying the will. This perception arose during a period of heightened racial and class conflict over Asian immigration into Western nations, and at a time when Enlightenment values of rationality, autonomy and individual agency were advancing. Most regular users of opiates were white middle-aged women, but public representations of opiate users during this period (the 1870s) circulated around the figure of the addicted Chinese immigrant as passive, corrupt and lazy.

Racist concerns even informed the discourse on route of drug administration: 'Eating and injecting opiates – the pattern most prevalent among affluent whites – was referred to as a disease, while the smoking of opium – a pattern associated with the Chinese – was labelled a vice' (2001: np). Of course, nowadays injecting is by and large a more stigmatised or vilified mode of drug administration than smoking or eating. Shifts in politics and the identification of HIV and hepatitis C as blood-borne viruses have played a major part in this change.

It is not possible to trace fully the development of the disease concept of addiction here, except to say it was by no means a linear process and involved periods in which medical approaches lost ground. More recently, however, a specific, highly refined medicalising approach, that of neuroscience, has gained influence. Helen Keane (2002) analyses this shift. She cites the adoption by the US National Institute of Drug Abuse (NIDA) of the principle that drug addiction is a disease of the brain. In this model, the drug addict's brain is understood to be materially different from that of the non-addict. According to the NIDA Director at the time of this shift, Alan Leshner, prolonged drug use throws a metaphorical 'switch' in the brain at which point the drug user becomes an addict. One NIDA article (Leshner 1999) explains it this way:

> NIDA research has demonstrated that using drugs repeatedly over time changes brain structure and function in fundamental and long-lasting ways that are part of the transition to compulsive abuse of drugs. Modern neuroscience techniques have enabled scientists to identify specific brain circuits involved in craving, euphoria, and other effects of addictive drugs. *NIDA Notes*, 16(5), 2001.

Keane describes this neuroscientific approach as merely an extreme example of the general oversimplifying trend operating in addiction science in that it is silent on the subjective experiences of drug users and also on the social context of drug use and addiction, not to mention the rest of the drug user's body beyond the brain. She goes on to demonstrate the fragility of the neuroscientific model, arguing that the imaging technologies it relies on do not offer the objective, scientific tools for diagnosing disease to which they lay claim. Rather, they are themselves dependent on prior social judgements of subjects as 'healthy and unhealthy ... not on the basis of abstract chemical or biological indicators, but on the *assessment of conduct*' (2002: 27).

Of course, it is the very claim to scientific objectivity that most appeals to scholars, health providers and policymakers who support the medicalisation of addiction, and to whom neuroscientific models can appeal. Advocates make a twofold argument: 1. science produces the most sound, reliable knowledge about drug use; and 2. this knowledge can be used to support measures – compassionate or merely pragmatic responses to drug use, such as the introduction of needle exchanges and medically supervised injecting facilities – that would otherwise be impossible to implement due to stigma and prejudice in relation to addiction. Put simply, the medicalisation of addiction is seen to provide a scientific explanation for what had previously been understood as a failure of the will, and, in line with Conrad and Schneider's argument about medicalisation in general, this scientisation has been regarded as destigmatising and progressive.

In contrast to this view, however, some scholars argue that the shift to a medical model of addiction has merely shifted the forms of stigmatisation in operation, rather than removed stigma altogether. As Brook and Stringer (2005) argue, where drug users are framed as diseased and in need of therapeutic intervention, and the drug itself is seen as virulently poisonous, it is clear that medicalising processes that frame drug use as a 'health problem' do not necessarily preclude moral judgements about either. From this point of view, the 'failure of the will' traditionally associated with addiction is actually institutionalised by medicine, crystallising, rather than disrupting, essentially arbitrary negative judgments about drug users.

This debate, its movement back and forth between notions of medicalisation as beneficial and as harmful, is not entirely unique (it shares parallels with debates on mental illness for instance) yet it distinguishes the meshed issues of addiction, injecting drug use and hepatitis C from other health issues such as cancer in obvious ways. As the first author (Suzanne Fraser) has argued elsewhere in collaboration with other authors (Fraser and valentine 2008, Moore and Fraser 2006, Roberts, valentine and Fraser 2009) people who inject drugs figure as less than fully rational subjects within Western liberal discursive contexts such as the clinical encounter. For these subjects, medicalisation simultaneously offers the prospect of acceptance as the 'merely sick', and this framing would appear to work consistently with a hepatitis C diagnosis, yet the particular emphasis it now puts on ideas of the agentic health consumer mean 'addicts' (framed as they are as passive and controlled by irrational forces) are never accepted as fully competent patients anyway. Clearly, both addiction and hepatitis C have been medicalised over time, but in rather different senses, and with different effects. The impact of this encounter between differing forms of medicalisation is partly the subject of this chapter. To begin laying out the terrain for closer consideration of this issue, we will draw from the foregoing discussion some key summary points.

Early proponents of the critique of medicalisation argued that medicine was often ineffective and productive of harmful side effects, and that its power and influence were not justified. They argued that medicalisation was actually a means of managing deviance. These perspectives were later subject to criticism as too negative and simplistic. Some later commentators argued that in earlier accounts the agency of patients had been ignored. Critics now acknowledge that medicine can improve lives, and that patients are increasingly included in medical decision-making processes, seen as able to manage their own health and make informed choices about medical procedures. This, it is noted, allows patients more control over their health but also imposes more responsibility. In short, accounts of the role of medicine have changed over time to become more ready to acknowledge the aspects of medicine that are effective, to see medicine as an intrinsic aspect of contemporary life, and to recognise that patients are (often a willing and active) part of the processes of medicalisation. How does this rather more complex picture of medicine operate in relation to addiction and hepatitis C? As was also spelt out above, addiction has its own particular history of medicalisation, and opinion on the merits of this process is mixed. What of the medical constitution of hepatitis C? A new disease has been named and has given a series of symptoms some legitimacy. Detection mechanisms, health advice and treatments for the disease have been developed. All this is surely to be welcomed. Yet as Chapter 1 began to suggest, it is possible to raise questions here, particularly when medical discourses of addiction and hepatitis C encounter each other – as the interviews informing this chapter will demonstrate. To help illuminate this issue, it is useful to turn to a set of terms recently developed in the context of the critique of medicalisation – those comprising Nikolas Rose's idea of biological citizenship.

From medicalisation to biological citizenship?

In his 2007 book *The Politics of Life Itself* (2007a), Rose makes the same point he puts forward in the debate covered above, in that he argues that a purely negative critical approach to biomedicine is inadequate. In his view we need to see biomedicine as a phenomenon by which we, in some ways willingly, are constituted, and this generates opportunities for experimentation and contestation (2007a: 39-40). Rose's work offers some specific insights into the production of hepatitis C and its subjects at the same time that it meshes with our broader concerns about the making of disease and the articulation of complexity. Mol, Law and Latour all remind us that phenomena are made in action, and that objects are always already multiple. Latour offers us the language to distinguish matters of concern from matters of fact, to render the ontology of disease more effectively. The biological citizens Rose tracks in his work are themselves phenomena made in action – as we will see, they are multiple: more than one but quite decidedly less than many in the limits of the resources, possibilities and options operating in and around them.

As we noted in the Introduction, Rose argues that health and illness are no longer simply polarised. Instead, we are expected to pursue self improvement continually. It is no longer acceptable to say, 'I am not ill, therefore I am well, and this is enough'. Instead, society encourages us to see ourselves as always open to somatic improvement, and always vulnerable to its opposite: ill health and physical decline. This perspective, Rose argues, along with the technologies developed in reflecting and promulgating it, have multiple effects: they open new avenues of both hope and fear in our lives.

According to Rose, biological citizenship emerges in the expectation that we must continually act to safeguard and enhance our health and our somatic integrity, combined with the expectation that we will do so voluntarily and as an expression of our true selves. Writing elsewhere with Paul Rabinow (2006), Rose argues that a new account of the relations between power and the body is required, one that exceeds the limitations of the now redundant notion of sovereign power for Western liberal democracies and can encompass the subtle ways in which citizens' participation and cooperation are secured. Drawing on Foucault's idea of biopower, Rabinow and Rose elaborate the notion of biopolitics, intended to understand politics and power without treating them as originating in the state. As they explain (2006: 199):

> Biopower, for Foucault, does not emerge from, or serve to support, a single power block, dominant group or set of interests.

This more diffuse model of power characterises Rose's approach to contemporary biomedicine and health in general.

Within the framework he spells out in *The Politics of Life Itself* are five pathways through which modes of biological citizenship are being expressed:

1. Molecularisation;
2. Optimisation;
3. Subjectification;
4. Somatic expertise;
5. Economics of vitality.

The argument being built in this chapter will focus on items 2 and 3, although all five pathways are relevant to the contemporary constitution of hepatitis C and its medical subjects. In relation to *optimisation*, Rose argues that the poles of health and illness have been augmented by interventions which 'seek to act in the present in order to secure the best possible future for those who are their subjects' (2006: 6). As we will see, hepatitis C-related medical interactions do just this, but readers addressed in this way respond to these imperatives in a particular range of registers. In relation to *subjectification*, Rose argues that human rights, duties and expectations are being reframed in terms of sickness, and more broadly, of 'life itself', that relations between individuals and medical authorities are being reorganised, and that subjects are increasingly expected to relate to themselves as 'somatic individuals' (2006: 6). In the process, they are expected to take responsibility for educating and reflecting on themselves, and for acting to enhance their health and wellbeing. As Rose (2006: 147) explains,

> The enactment of such responsible behaviours has become routine and expected, built in to public health measures, producing new types of problematic persons – those who refuse to identify themselves with this responsible community of biological citizens.

These shifts are creating a new somatic ethics which constitutes values for living along explicitly corporeal lines. These values, Rose argues, can be framed in terms of Immanuel Kant's famous three questions: What can I know? What must I do? What may I hope? Taken together, these three questions encapsulate the key reflexive issues for contemporary biological citizens. Again, as we will see, this emphasis on the corporeal, on understanding the self as primarily enacted via agential decision-making around health management and the pre-emption of somatic problems, is also applied to people who inject drugs diagnosed with hepatitis C, with highly mixed effects and implications.[2]

What Can I Know? What Must I Do?

We have already observed that contemporary health promotion aimed at people who inject drugs enacts neo-liberal norms of individual responsibility, even as the target audience constitutes one of the most structurally disadvantaged populations within Western liberal democracies (Fraser 2004). The literature's focus on self-care and individual responsibility renders it a significant expression of biological citizenship as characterised by Rose. Likewise, the drug treatment clinical encounter also enacts norms of individual responsibility and self-care, although these are much less consistently applied, and the trust and respect they imply is

---

2   Orsini (2008) has also linked hepatitis C and Rose's concepts in an article focusing on political contestation as biological citizenship. The analysis conducted in this chapter differs from Orsini's work in that we draw a much broader definition of biological citizenship from Rose and colleagues' work and aim to consider alongside macro-level dynamics of power and contestation the subtle, self-constituting aspects of these new modes of self-body engagement.

less consistently bestowed (Roberts, valentine and Fraser 2009). The interviews analysed here make clear that people who inject drugs regularly grapple with these powerful injunctions around responsibility and self-care in hepatitis C education literature and the clinical encounter, particularly in relation to awareness of new hepatitis C-related information about transmission, health and treatment options. In certain ways, they are invited, and expected, to behave as modern biological citizens. How do these interview participants respond to these injunctions? What are we to make of their responses? What are the implications of their responses for notions of biological citizenship and for the debate around the advantages and disadvantages of medicalisation in this context? These questions will be tackled below. In doing so, the chapter will move beyond what have now become well-established observations about the responsibilisation of drug users. It aims to consider what can be read in some respects as the next set of pressing issues: how, exactly, this responsibilisation relates to notions of drug addiction, to the management of hepatitis C as chronic illness, and ultimately to the very particular politics surrounding the medicalisation of addiction.

As noted at the outset, this chapter was initially prompted by a trend visible in the interview data indicating that some people who inject drugs do not pursue information and advice about hepatitis C after diagnosis. The information initially accessed in the diagnostic clinical encounter sometimes forms the only knowledge acquired, and the only basis on which health and self-care decisions are made, for many years following diagnosis. This response to diagnosis is evident in the statements of many of the interview participants. Here we will present as case studies three participants who share this initial response, but who diverge in their experiences across time: Andy, Giuseppe and Stacey. Together these participants' trajectories of engagement with hepatitis C medical and health promotion knowledges broadly reflect the different engagement 'careers' of the interview participants as a group.

Andy

Andy is a 29-year old Anglo-Australian resident of a northern suburb of Melbourne. When asked about how closely he follows developments in knowledge about hepatitis C, he explains that he does not 'really bother' to pick up and read the new literature made available in the needle exchange (NSP) he regularly visits. Diagnosed in prison in 1999, and reportedly asymptomatic since then, Andy was given some information at the time, but describes having read very little since. His hepatitis C is not altogether forgotten however. It comes up at times in consultations with the general practitioner (GP) who prescribes Andy's methadone. According to Andy, the GP:

> want(s) me to either get off the methadone or, you know, be stable or something, and then look at options for the treatment or whatever of my hepatitis C.

Andy is by no means enthusiastic about undergoing treatment. He regards himself as 'unstable' in that his housing is unsatisfactory. As he puts it,

> I share with people I don't really like and like, stress levels are high [...] so I don't want to go through all that while I'm already on edge [...]

Presumably, in using the word 'unstable' (which comes up several times as he describes himself) Andy is also referring to the fact that he continues to inject heroin. This is one of the standard meanings of the expression within opioid pharmacotherapy treatment in Australia.

Later on in the interview Andy reiterates his views about information, explaining that he sees little point in keeping up to date on hepatitis C until he is in a position to act on this information.

> Oh, to tell the truth, unless I actually go right ahead and do something about it and get treatment and everything, it's pointless looking at a pamphlet [...] I want everything else to be right before I look into that stage of my life, you know.

Interestingly, Andy goes so far as to nominate possession of a job as a necessary precondition for undergoing treatment. Given that the side effects of treatment can be severe, many people on treatment choose to minimise paid employment during the six or twelve months over which they are treated. Andy is aware that treatment causes serious side effects, so it seems his nomination of a job relates to concerns other than the basic living and drug use conditions that would improve his experience of treatment. What are they? This question will be revisited at the end of this section.

More broadly, Andy equates action with undergoing treatment, although he does act in other ways in relation to hepatitis C, for example, he minimises his consumption of alcohol as originally advised when diagnosed (although it must be noted that his intake is still substantial by comparison with current Australian guidelines), and pays attention to injecting equipment and the need to avoid sharing needles. In this respect Andy demonstrates awareness of some of the key features of current prevention injunctions in relation to hepatitis C. In other respects, however, his engagement with these injunctions is minimal. He has, for instance, no idea which hepatitis C genotype he carries, and therefore what odds of clearing the disease would accompany treatment for him. In fact, he has little understanding of how genotype is established and how to go about accessing that information. Hepatitis C genotype has become more widely understood among hepatitis C positive people over the last ten years. It seems that the information Andy accessed on diagnosis has remained with him, while further refinements of this information, and new areas of knowledge and advice, are largely absent.

Giuseppe

Giuseppe is another participant who reported a long period of inactivity in relation to hepatitis C awareness after diagnosis. A 41-year old Italian-Australian resident of inner Melbourne, Giuseppe contracted hepatitis C prior to 1989 when it was still referred to as non-A, non-B hepatitis. He is a regular heroin consumer and methadone client. Giuseppe's account of his interest in hepatitis C and his own diagnosis differs from Andy's in some important respects in that over time Giuseppe has become increasingly involved in his health and has developed a highly reflexive relationship to the issues thrown up by his hepatitis C. The perspective he offers on the reasons for his seroconversion to hepatitis C positive status provides a useful example of this reflexivity, in that he expresses some ambivalence about the role of individual agency and responsibility in the event. When asked whether, at the time that he contracted hepatitis C, he felt he had any real option to protect himself from infection, he responds as follows:

> I felt, well, at the time we didn't. But that can be a cop out too […] 'cause I didn't feel comfortable, or I didn't do enough work trying to get clean fits. That's my fault. Even though they weren't as widely available, and they asked more questions at the time, that was my fault that I didn't do what I had to do to get them. And I was happier to look under rock number five behind house forty where the creek is and get the fit from under there.

Here Giuseppe is arguing that although the structural circumstances surrounding the distribution of needles and syringes were significantly more constrained at the time than they are now, he could have made a more concerted effort to access clean equipment and to stay hepatitis C-free. His comments are directly followed by this exchange, which partly refers to the common desire to avoid NSPs as a means of keeping injecting practice secret:

> **Interviewer:** And be anonymous?
>
> **Giuseppe:** Yeah, exactly, that's exactly right. Almost anonymous from myself.

This final statement takes the interviewer's educated guess about Giuseppe's motives for reusing injecting equipment and adds an insightful twist, one that gestures towards a reflexivity highly congruent with contemporary features of biological citizenship. Giuseppe indicates that he has abandoned his prior desire to explicitly avoid self knowledge, and instead adopted the proper biocitizen's obligatory mode of rational, critical engagement with the self.

Indeed, prior to these comments, Giuseppe engages in the following exchange with the interviewer:

> **Interviewer:** Okay […] like, why did you decide to go on treatment at that point?

Giuseppe: I suppose I felt like I owed it to myself. I think I owed it to myself.

Interviewer: Can you tell me a bit more about that?

Giuseppe: Don't you have a relationship with yourself?

Interviewer: Yeah.

Giuseppe: I have and, like I said to you earlier, I felt like I let myself down by getting, by contracting, the virus. And I thought it was a chance to redeem myself.

In all these statements Giuseppe differs from Andy in that he reports an active engagement with his hepatitis C as an aspect of his identity and as a function of his reflexive and self-regulating capacities. He expresses an active ethical relationship with himself through the phenomenon of disease. This is not to say Andy lacks an ethical relationship with himself. In the course of his interview, however, this relationship is not expressed via the trope of disease. Both Andy and Giuseppe also report having reduced their alcohol intake after diagnosis, and limiting or eliminating the sharing of injecting equipment as well. In this respect they both reportedly initially followed public health injunctions. Yet at a particular point their parallel paths diverged abruptly. Giuseppe is explicit about the events that contributed to the changes he underwent: he describes a social worker who visited the rooming house in which he was living and who encouraged him to address his hepatitis C via a program offered through a Melbourne clinic. This encounter resulted in improved housing and an introduction to treatment services.

In relation to this introduction, Giuseppe makes a vivid statement about the meaning of treatment for him. He begins by describing the clinician he encountered and then draws the discussion around to his own decision-making process:

Giuseppe: The American dude, he was a bit of an evangelist sort of, and he was really, had a really loud voice, and he was a little bit intimidating. Not intimidating in a scary way, just I felt like he was carrying on a little bit.

Interviewer: What do you mean?

Giuseppe: 'Oh, come on, you can't keep living like this'. And 'cause I was telling him, look, he's going, 'you know you're going to have to [have treatment, it's] the best chance for you to be successful', 'cause I didn't want to go through it and it not to work [...]

Giuseppe: He saw heaps of people, like people that [were] like in and out of gaol, that had kids, responsibilities. I didn't have that, I didn't have the kids, I didn't have the gaol, I'd just got housing [problems]. So, I had housing [resolved now]. You know, all that sort of, tenuous sort of situation of, you could be sleeping in the park or whatever, wasn't happening no more, that was fixed up. So I thought, 'well I suppose this is the next step to being a citizen' type thing.

Interviewer: Can you tell me a bit more about that? What do you mean 'being a citizen'?

Giuseppe: Oh, you know, more conventional, having a more conventional life.

The steps towards citizenship Giuseppe describes also included agreeing to go on methadone maintenance treatment for his injecting drug use. It is clear the decision to do this was not lightly made. Giuseppe describes a drawn-out process in which the hepatitis C clinician cajoled him into methadone maintenance treatment despite significant misgivings on Giuseppe's part. In short, Giuseppe reports that he was not able to access treatment for hepatitis C until he also agreed to participate in methadone maintenance treatment first. In addition he reports having to attend group therapy meetings:

Yeah, the social worker [...] got me in touch with [peer treatment support worker], and she came and picked us up and we went down to a support group meeting, and I went there for about, almost a year before they started to consider me seriously for treatment.

Giuseppe describes this period prior to entering hepatitis C treatment as one in which he was stalled by the clinician as he attempted to find ways of satisfying the expectation of 'stability'. Giuseppe explains his hesitancy to commence methadone treatment as the result of prior negative experiences with the program and a fear of finding himself stuck on it indefinitely. In fact, he proposed being prescribed other medication such as codeine or morphine as a means of reducing his heroin use: 'something else, anything else, but I don't want to go back, I don't want methadone'.

Ultimately, according to Giuseppe, he acquiesced to expectations that he take methadone, and only then accessed hepatitis C treatment. At the time of interview he was still on methadone maintenance treatment, and had yet to hear whether the six months of hepatitis C treatment he had completed had been a success. As with the specific characteristics of Andy's relationship to his hepatitis C, we will return to the details of Giuseppe's story at the end of the section. In the meantime, we will introduce a third interview participant, whose approach to her health differs again from the two discussed so far.

Stacey

Stacey is a 24-year old woman of Eastern European heritage living in an outer south-eastern suburb of Melbourne. Stacey was diagnosed with hepatitis C in early adolescence and considers her seroconversion to be the result of a needle stick injury (although there is ambiguity in her interview about this as it is unclear whether she had also been sharing injecting equipment at the time.) For Stacey, accepting her diagnosis took some time. As with some other interview participants, Stacey needed more than one test and more than one clinical encounter in which she was diagnosed before she accepted the information. As she explains (in an extract also quoted in Chapter 3):

> **Stacey:** [The first doctor] told me and I stormed out, I didn't want to talk to him. I cracked the shits, I thought he was lying so I went to another doctor, he said the same thing and I stormed out. And then I went and spoke to my drug and alcohol counsellors, that's how I found out about it, like what it does and I got the book and all that kind of crap about it. And yeah, I looked right into it.

> **Interviewer:** Why did you crack the shits?

> **Stacey:** 'Cause I thought he was lying to me, to be honest with you. I'm like, 'no, bullshit, I couldn't't', I just thought it wasn't possible, from stepping on a syringe. 'Get fucked', you know what I mean, that's what I thought […] And I walked down to another doctor, got a blood test and he said the same thing. I went, 'all right, thanks' and walked out. I don't like doctors, I don't go to doctors […] I can't handle them. They tell you too much, they think they know you, but as far as I'm concerned you know your body better than anyone.

As does Giuseppe in his comments about methadone, Stacey indicates a significant amount of suspicion towards medicine. Indeed, her doubts are so pronounced she requires multiple tests and multiple clinical encounters with different practitioners before she is convinced of her diagnosis.

Like both Andy and Giuseppe, diagnosis was followed by a long period in which Stacey paid little or no attention to her hepatitis C. As she puts it:

> […] when I found out, I was like, 'I don't care' and if I had to [share injecting equipment], and a friend goes 'I've got hep C', I'm like 'oh, I've got it already, so it's not like I'm going to catch it again'. And yeah, [that's] until probably about seven years ago [when] I stopped using, stopped sharing and all that kind of stuff […]

Later Stacey explains her reaction further:

> **Stacey:** At the time I didn't care, to be honest. I was too busy in the drug scene. I was too busy making friends, partying, taking drugs, I didn't really give a shit to be honest. I didn't even think about it.

> **Interviewer:** And do you give a shit now?

Stacey: Oh yeah. About, up to about, what was it, five, maybe six, years ago I started really looking after myself.

Stacey's change in perspective was initiated by a health scare in which she experienced a fainting episode and a hospital stay, and took a liver function test with worrying results. She then became motivated to increase her knowledge of hepatitis C, and did so while serving a subsequent prison sentence. But this did not mean she developed a more trusting or collaborative approach to medicine. Indeed, she describes her increased level of education as a means of resisting medicine's arrogance:

> [...] when I was in gaol all I did was read. Like I know my law, I know my doctors, I know everything, I made sure I knew everything so that if someone turned around and said something I could go, 'no, fuck you, I know that that's wrong'.

Overall, Stacey is highly wary of those involved in the hepatitis C medical sector. She views them as largely motivated by the prospect of individual gain:

> I know a lot of professionals who are about hep C and don't really care, they're only in it because it's getting so big that they can make money on it. Like, they can make a living from it [...]

Alongside this rather negative view of medical practitioners appears to run a relatively extensive engagement with hepatitis C-related medical information. Unlike many of the interview participants, Stacey now keeps a library of publications on hepatitis C. Again, however, it is worth emphasising that this engagement with information of medical origin does not draw her into a warmer or more cooperative relationship with the healthcare system:

> It's just all the same thing, everywhere you go, just the same crap, they treat you like you're an idiot, like you don't know nothing about it, and at the end of the day I probably know more than them. Because I've [...] made sure I know about it. And when you tell them that they go, 'well, you can't know everything'. And it's like, 'do you want to come to my house, I've got fricking, a bookshelf, one shelf just full of books on hep C, so'.

This literature and the confidence it appears to inspire in Stacey is also augmented by regular and extensive internet searches, although it should be noted that Stacey does not necessarily have a reliable grasp of hepatitis C, given she states she is currently infected with an extremely unlikely total of seven genotypes. Does her active pursuit of health knowledge and understanding mean Stacey is an exemplary biological citizen? Somehow her attitudes render an answer in the affirmative problematic.

There are clearly many variations in the ways individuals with hepatitis C interviewed for the study described here responded to diagnosis, and engaged with or ignored information about their condition. The three case studies all indicate a lengthy absence of engagement directly after diagnosis, but motivations for this absence, and the events subsequent to it, vary enormously. Ultimately, Andy remains alienated from medical responses to hepatitis C. Giuseppe has engaged thoroughly with the options medicine provides, though not entirely willingly. And Stacey pursues knowledge actively, while maintaining a highly skeptical relationship to medical practitioners. What do these responses say about biomedicine and biological citizenship?

Despite their variety, all three case studies point to a key issue in relation to medicine. That is that despite the tendency to take as an article of faith the value of medicalisation in countering stigma and opening the way for action to ameliorate the effects of addiction and related health problems, the medicalisation of phenomena such as illness does not, in itself, guarantee any particular favourable outcome (Brownscombe 2004). Indeed, as the material presented above suggests, the medicalisation of hepatitis C (and, in Giuseppe's case, of addiction – via the injunction to seek treatment for his heroin use) is of little or no use to participants on its own. In the case of Andy, that addiction has been medicalised is largely meaningless. Andy is profoundly socially and materially disadvantaged, and may always have been (that is, prior to his drug use). His disadvantage operates as a powerful obstacle to engagement with hepatitis C-related information and health-related activity. In this respect, he sits somewhat outside Rose's notion of biological citizenship, although it is true that he expresses an awareness of health injunctions and has reportedly followed some of these to some degree. It seems that for Andy, further engagement with corporeal modes of enacting a responsible, citizen-like self depends on the presence of factors that themselves are markers of *prior* citizenship status: decent housing, employment and so on. In no sense, that is, does Andy's limited engagement with medicine or his health appear to confer a sense of participation, social or political engagement or belonging that might be expected in relation to biological citizenship. In no sense does Andy appear to embrace the opportunities associated with biological citizenship, in which, to use Rose's words (2007a: 141):

> [i]ndividuals are actively engaged with biological explanations and forming novel relations with scientific or medical authorities in the process of caring for, and about, health.

Instead, biological citizenship's injunctions, unattainable and alien as they are to Andy, seem mainly to underline his exclusion.

In Giuseppe's case a similar set of circumstances prevailed until he came into contact with a particularly active and effective social worker who led him to engage with health and medicine in new ways. This led to a relationship with another highly active healthcare professional whose strenuous recommendations around methadone maintenance treatment, hepatitis C treatment and the possibility of a new life took some time to sink in, but ultimately influenced Giuseppe to view himself and act in new ways. In the process of recounting this development, Giuseppe expresses a highly reflexive perspective and an absolutely overt awareness of the opportunity for belonging, or citizenship, that enacting mainstream forms of health can confer. In this sense, Giuseppe has become an exemplary biological citizen – indeed, his ongoing critical relationship with medicine only cements this new role in that modern health subjects are expected to maintain a degree of caution and autonomy in their decision-making about health. Of course, the highly intrusive role Giuseppe's treatment clinician played in his deliberations about treatment belies this ideal. According to Giuseppe's account, his actions and opinions are very actively 'managed' by healthcare professionals who, in this context at least, appear to view vigorous promotion of treatment regimes part of the role of medicine. Obviously, this does not coincide with contemporary mainstream models of the clinical encounter which prioritise patient independence via the notion of the individual's right and responsibility to make rational, informed decisions based on information provided by practitioners, but not subject to undue influence by practitioners. Giuseppe's status as an injecting drug user, and an 'addict' according to White's criteria listed earlier (craving, tolerance, loss of volitional control over consumption, negative consequences of consumption and so on), are likely to play an important part in this dynamic. Where Giuseppe is understood to be suffering from a disease of the will, unable to reflect accurately on himself or act effectively to solve his problems, he becomes subject to a clinician/patient relationship rather different from that promoted through contemporary rationalist ideals. This alternative relationship is not new to medicine: it recalls older models based on a paternalistic form of fiduciary duty.

What of Stacey? Her active engagement with medical literature – her belief that knowledge constitutes power in the clinical encounter conforms closely to contemporary norms of patient engagement. Yet her highly antagonistic relationship to medical practitioners, and her negative view of the motives of those working in the sector does not. Modern patients are expected to see their healthcare providers as partners in health, partners who provide considered, unbiased information and advice, upon which considered and sensible health decisions are made. This is the role medicine idealises, one partly built on the progressivist heroic ideal demonstrated in Chapter 1. For Stacey, literature fulfils this role while people do not.

Stacey's unique approach to her health goes further in that she presents her time in gaol as an opportunity to increase what might be called her 'cultural capital' (Bourdieu 1986). Along with health information, she also gathered information on her legal rights. The shift in power Stacey sees as having been gained with this new knowledge is interesting to consider in the context of biological citizenship. Stacey is of course not alone in having viewed gaol time as affording the chance to 'improve' herself. Yet Stacey does not follow the fabled path of redemption here. She remains engaged in illicit drug use and maintains significant links to organised crime. She does not develop a cooperative relationship with medicine. Thus she does not altogether embody the ideal Rose points to in his earlier (2000: 489) article on these issues, co-authored with Carlos Novas:

> The patient is to become skilled, prudent and active, an ally of the doctor, a proto-professional...

Yes, Stacey is perhaps able to act as a relatively autonomous agent in navigating the clinical encounter. It is, however, rather difficult to frame her as an ally of the doctor. Equally, while her general approach to her health is obviously active, it does not register convincingly, at least to these observers, as 'prudent' or 'proto-professional'. Does Stacey rely on the rational in her decision making? Here it is worth quoting her reaction to the advice encountered in the literature:

> **Interviewer:** So you've pretty much followed the advice in the books?
>
> **Stacey:** Oh yeah, finding out, oh, certain advice I've followed. What I've agreed with I've followed. If I read something and I don't agree with it, I'm stubborn, I won't do it, even if it's right, I won't do it.
>
> **Interviewer:** Yeah? Which bits? Do you remember some of the stuff that you haven't agreed with?
>
> **Stacey:** Oh some of the food, like they tell you to eat avocados and shit like that. I hate avocado, but they tell you that it's really, really good for your liver, and it's like, 'yeah, well I don't give a shit what's really good for my liver at the moment, I don't like it, I'm not eating it'. Do you know what I mean? Like rest, like how they tell you should have, what seven, I think it was ten hours sleep, and it's like, 'get fucked, I've got a life, how am I going to get ten hours' sleep?' My bloke's got to wake up at five to go to work, we're lucky to get six to eight hours a night. Like, no one can get ten hours' sleep, do you know what I mean? Hep C or no hep C, they've got to be dreaming.

Not only is Stacey pointing, here, to the gap between advice given and the realities of her life, she is also expressing a rather complicated, and certainly not ideally rational, relationship to the advice. On the one hand, she says that if she agrees with advice, she will follow it. On the other, she says she is stubborn, and might refuse to follow advice even when she knows it is correct.

Does Stacey's approach to health and medicine, her history and her relationship to knowledge constitute biological citizenship according to the broad parameters proposed by Rose and others? Does Stacey build a self, and access a platform of legitimacy as a citizen, from the opportunities and prohibitions generated by the increasing focus on health, on the responsible, self-regulating pre-emption of illness and the concomitant blurring of the line between sickness and wellness? Or does she in some senses constitute one of those in the new category of the non-compliant Rose identifies (2007a: 147); a new type of problematic person – one who refuses to align herself properly with the responsible community of biological citizens? Yes and no, it seems. These are questions we can ask of all three participants described here. Before we too hastily begin diagnosing these participants, however, there are several observations that need to be revisited about the context of these questions.

The first relates to the issue of whether Andy, Giuseppe and Stacey exhibit the obligatory degree of active, rational and prudent self-management in relation to their health. All three have considered undergoing treatment for hepatitis C, but only Giuseppe has done so. Is undergoing treatment for hepatitis C in itself active, rational and prudent? Despite highly variable success rates for combination interferon and ribavirin) treatment (as high as 80-90 per cent for genotypes 2 and 3 across 24 weeks of treatment, and as low as 40-45 per cent for genotypes 1 and 4 across 48 weeks of treatment (Department of Health and Ageing 2008: 134), many people are encouraged to try treatment, or, as with Giuseppe, to work towards establishing the conditions under which it would be conceivable. How should this encouragement be viewed? Even where treatment is successful and a sustained virological response (clearance) is achieved, some patients continue to feel unwell. The impact on work, relationships and quality of life during treatment is severe. Thus, while clinicians working in a broad public health framework that sees widespread treatment as part of a necessary response to high incidence rates may be inclined to recommend treatment, and while it can be argued that embarking on it constitutes agentic activity and self-management, it is not necessarily a rational or prudent response. Stacey, for example, provides a powerful account of the grounds on which she has resisted treatment. Her past partner had been on combination interferon and ribavirin for two months, and had a history of depression:

> I walked in the bathroom and he was hanging from the roof, 'cause we had rafters in the bathroom, and he was half dead. Like I got him, cut him down and he had a like, boomp, boomp [heartbeat], and it was almost stopped and I called the ambos and shit like that. So yeah, so that's why I refused to get on it, I saw what happened to him […] Like, he's still got scars from it. So yeah, no, fuck that, I don't want to get on …

Indeed, given uncertain rates of success and uncertain outcomes in terms of wellness, but a high likelihood of serious side effects, there is an important sense in which choosing to undergo treatment constitutes a significant risk. Of course, the idea that medical treatments or procedures carry an element of risk is not a new one. Yet it has particular salience for those routinely framed as illegitimate risk takers, as lacking prudence and as subject to the agency of substance and lacking agency or will of their own. For these uniquely located subjects, the enactment of biological citizenship is especially complex, and not a little complicated by the subtle hypocrisies of normalisation.

Also necessary to consider here is the broader status of medicalisation in relation to addiction and hepatitis C. As all three case studies suggest, there is an important sense in which the medicalisation of addiction on its own can be of only limited benefit to individual drug users' lives, and that in any case it has only partially been achieved in Western liberal democracies. Two of the three participants described here had spent time in gaol. Evidently, suffering from the 'brain disease' of addiction has not exempted them from responsibility and punishment for their behaviour. Indeed, problems associated with drug use are in many cases addressed, and largely punitively, by the criminal justice system rather than the health system. Having the 'disease' of addiction means Andy can access methadone maintenance treatment, but the benefits of this to his daily life are also limited, especially given the treatment model is itself highly inflected by criminal justice considerations which impact on key issues such as the availability of takeaway doses (Fraser and valentine 2008). Thus Andy remains heavily marginalised. Giuseppe has also engaged with medical responses to injecting drug use and hepatitis C in that he is also, albeit reluctantly, on methadone, and has undergone six months of treatment for hepatitis C. In Giuseppe's case, it was a new engagement with non-clinical professionals, mainly social workers and peer support workers, that initially led him to take this direction. Interpersonal contact with workers offering new forms of support and resourcing made a profound difference for Giuseppe. In this respect, and despite a common tendency to wish it so, medicalisation alone does not, of course, solve complex social problems. Indeed, given that the outcome of Giuseppe's hepatitis C treatment was at the time of interview still unknown, given he reports it to have been severely disruptive to his life, and given he is not really happy to be on methadone, the benefits of medicalisation for this hepatitis C-positive injecting drug user are at this stage not altogether clear.

Related to this point is the need to consider how addiction complicates normative expectations about the autonomous subject of health. The traditional critique of medicalisation, as was noted earlier, holds that medicine can be ineffective, can produce harmful side effects, possesses an unjustifiably high degree of power and influence, and is actually a means of managing deviance. As was also noted, these perspectives were later subject to criticism as too negative and simplistic and as failing to recognise that patients are often a willing and active part of the processes of medicalisation. In that material and social disadvantage is found in much higher concentrations among people who inject drugs than in the general population, and the 'addict' label erodes the subject's status as rational and self-managing, some of the current analyses of medicalisation that emphasise the active, highly informed, deliberative role of patients in expanding (usually beneficial) medical options are less convincing for this group. In some important respects, it must be said, the stories of Andy, Giuseppe and Stacey align with the former approach to medicine more than the latter in that each is subject to significant structural disadvantage, has had little or no say in the design or implementation of treatments available to them, and is yet to experience an unambiguously positive outcome from these treatments.

Of equally uncertain relevance to this group, the current, less negative, approach describes an additional relationship that has developed alongside the notion of the autonomous patient in partnership with the clinician: that *between patients themselves*, when, as Rose (2007a: 134) argues, biological citizenship takes the form of a 'collectivising' moment. According to Rose (2007a: 149):

> Biological citizenship requires those with investments in their biology to become political.

As Rose notes, the consumer health movement has both emerged from the shift to a focus on individual action and responsibility and contributed to it. A medical diagnosis can introduce individuals to a highly active, highly politically savvy network of patient advocates capable of promoting their group interests, both within medicine and more broadly in the political and policy realms. While there is no doubt that recent years have seen an expansion in peer advocacy activity among people who inject drugs, and the establishment of related advocacy organisations receiving some government-funding, and while similar activity does occur in the specific area of hepatitis C,[3] the model of the politically active patient, uniting with other patients, often over the internet, to campaign for extra funding, new treatment options and other health benefits, is a poor fit for the vast majority affected by hepatitis C. Even in the area of methadone maintenance treatment, another medical focus for people who inject drugs, there is little in the way of a coordinated political engagement among patients – in spite of the fact that treatment involves almost daily congregation at dosing points (Fraser, valentine and Roberts 2009; Fraser and valentine 2008). There are many reasons for this relatively low level of political organising, including the difficulties involved in uniting around such a heavily stigmatised, legally marginal identity for the purposes of rights-based claims making, and the material disadvantage that characterises this population (Orsini 2008). Nevertheless, individual examples of this kind of response do exist. Giuseppe, for instance, reports moving into a hepatitis C-related advocacy role via his recently completed welfare training.

In effect, then, while the feature of biological citizenship that Rose elucidates here – that of active political engagement around biology – can be seen in some initiatives, it is neither widespread among nor readily available to people with hepatitis C. Of course, Rose does not assume that this form of biological citizenship is evenly distributed. He recognises that Western conventions around active medical subjecthood are not found in all parts of the world when he notes

---

3   These include organisations such as Australia's peak body for illicit drug user organisations, AIVL (the Australian Injecting and Illicit Drug Users League), and the state-based hepatitis C councils, which incorporate significant levels of peer involvement.

that (2007a: 147): 'such forms of biosociality ... have no visible presence in many geographical regions'. Yet, as the case of hepatitis C suggests, we do not need to look so far afield geographically to observe the limits of biological citizenship. People who inject drugs cannot be the sole health constituency in Western liberal democracies that, despite vigorous interpellations, is only marginally engaged with contemporary medical ideals of patient responsibility and activity and their rewards. What does this marginality mean for the observations Rose and others have made about biological citizenship? Do contemporary injunctions actually lack bite? Is biological citizenship a myth, or, at best, a phenomenon of the educated and affluent?

It would not do to oversimplify biological citizenship here. While it is important to consider how 'portable' (in Law's terms) are its injunctions and norms across social and economic difference, and to question whether all subjects of contemporary health are addressed in the same ways and enjoy the same validation in enacting biological citizenship, it is also necessary to see the features of biological citizenship as multiple and at times discontinuous and contradictory. Hepatitis C positive people who inject drugs find themselves medicalised in ways that are profoundly paradoxical. They are at times encouraged to exercise agency in their pursuit of health, at others 'managed' in ways that seek to circumvent their putatively pathological agency. They are marginalised as risk-takers yet invited to court risk (through treatment). Above all, and perhaps this goes without saying, the 'somatic individuality' we might argue they enact in consuming drugs, in acting on their corporeal selves via the mechanism of drugs (in flicking, even, the neurological 'switch' constructed by NIDA), disqualifies rather than qualifies them as biological citizens. For these health subjects, the expectations and the rewards of biological citizenship are elusive and uncertain. Yet this is also the case, to different degrees, for all subjects of contemporary health. Menopausal women, for instance, also register as rather less than fully rational in medical representations and practice (Roberts, valentine and Fraser 2009). This shapes the ways they are addressed and the extent to which their health generates opportunities and resources for political and social belonging. Clearly we need to approach this phenomenon flexibly, and yet the points at which it fits least are highly significant, and so should not be overlooked.

Conclusion: What may [we] hope?

To extend, perhaps indefinitely, the hesitation in 'diagnosing' hepatitis C-positive people who inject drugs that marked the beginning of the foregoing series of observations, then, we want to conclude that the key to progress on hepatitis C prevention and harm reduction priorities lies not so much in continually searching out new ways of 'understanding' or 'explaining' or 'improving' these health subjects' decisions and actions. Instead it might better be served by focusing more consistently on the gaps and points of poor fit *between* contemporary discursive dynamics of biological citizenship and particular health subjects. Such gaps, we contend, allow crucial insights about the intersections of health, privilege and reason in Western liberal democracies. Shifting the focus in this way presents questions ultimately more pressing that those referred to earlier (asking whether hepatitis C-positive people who inject drugs constitute biological citizens, asking whether they succeed in enacting the expected attributes of rationality, responsibility and reflexivity and so on). Why? Because questions about injecting drug using subjects are asked repeatedly, almost compulsively it might be said, while questions about the biopolitical circumstances and forces through which they are constituted are asked relatively rarely. What is it, exactly, these subjects are asked to enact? Are these expectations themselves rational, responsible and reflexively constituted, or do they merely express un-thought out Enlightenment norms and assumptions about activity, reason and science? What happens when hepatitis C-positive people who inject drugs are seen both as flawed, addicted subjects for whom rationality and self-management are but fantasies, and as reasoning health consumers in possession of the necessary resources and ambition to choose onerous health measures and treatment regimes as an expression of their agency and efficacy? Even more pressingly, what should we make of these measures and regimes themselves? How 'rational' and 'reasonable' indeed are they? Do they represent prudence or risk taking, or both? Do their 'benefits outweigh their risks' (to use the quintessential contemporary parlance)? What does it mean to recommend and even to enjoin behaviours, or to offer health measures and regimes, that may, as we saw in Chapter 1, be discredited or superseded within a few years? Who is it, in short, acting on faith, compelled by expectations and desires, hopes and fears? Is it the targeted and thus constituted biological citizens, or is it also those working in public health and medicine who help generate the discourses that in turn shape these citizens? Both it would seem, and in this sense the recommendations, injunctions and obligations generated must be examined as carefully and with an eye to the operations of the non-rational as those of individual health consumers.

Hepatitis C-positive people who inject drugs are constantly invited to navigate Kant's three questions – to engage, in the process, in a complex and demanding relationship with themselves. But there is a corresponding need to turn these questions around and apply them to medicine and public health as well, and to likewise expect them to engage in a relationship with themselves and their ambitions. What can *they* know? What must *they* do? What may *they* hope? If contemporary society has transformed health into a key resource for social and political belonging, medicine and public health's responsibilities for the most marginalised and disadvantaged are even more substantial than conceived to date. And their expectations and demands must be thought accordingly. This includes the notion that an uncritical alignment with 'medicalisation' will serve the interests of those labelled addicts into the future of biological citizenship. With all its injunctions to reason, responsibility and self-management, biological citizenship would seem to always already disqualify hepatitis C-positive people who inject drugs from legitimacy and the rewards attendant on this mode of engagement with health and medicine. Given the acknowledged centrality of the social and political in health outcomes, there is an urgent need to conceive effective responses to hepatitis C multiply, certainly beyond medical measures alone. But how to do this strategically and effectively? This, perhaps ironically, perhaps fittingly, is an opening for yet another enactment of biological citizenship: one for which those of us with professional, scholarly and political stakes in the debate as well as the inevitable biological ones, are also 'responsible'.

Chapter 5

From Centre to Periphery: The Ethics and Politics of Treatment

'...the promise of treatment is that you will be transformed in some way'.

(Ellen, female, 58 years)

'...where does the interferon stop and I begin?'

(Giuseppe, male, 41 years)

This chapter examines individual pathways into and experiences of medical treatment for hepatitis C. It picks up on several of the themes touched on in the previous chapter, where we began to consider some of the ways in which treatment comes to be offered to individuals living with hepatitis C and their various responses to these offers. In the sections that follow we critically evaluate claims about the nature and function of treatment further, drawing on interviews we discussed in Chapter 4. This chapter again considers some questions about the pathway into treatment, but this time with a specific focus on how these pathways perform subjects. In addition, the chapter considers a new area: how people who have undergone treatment experience that treatment and what, for these people, treatment *does*. The central premise of the chapter is that medicine acts upon, performs and transforms its subjects. We argue that it does so in three main ways: by producing them as 'ordered' and/or 'chaotic', as 'successful' and/or 'failed', and through the 'despair' associated with treatment. Treatment, we argue, performs its subjects in familiar, often normative, ways. This has important implications for the lived experience of people with hepatitis C, for our understandings of drug use and for people who inject drugs.

The chapter also builds on some of the observations made in Chapter 1, and our quasispecies epistemology. As we will see, several of the features we identified as comprising a quasispecies epistemology are relevant to this discussion. These are, first, the notion of error and chaos as productive – as entailed in, rather than antithetical to, order; and secondly, the significance of constant motion. In this chapter we consider how questions of order, chaos and constant motion feature in relation to hepatitis C treatment. The chapter extends our previous observations by considering some of the novel ways in which order, chaos and constant motion produce new phenomena in and through treatment. In particular, we look at the way they produce subjects. Throughout this book we have drawn on Annemarie Mol's work to think through disease, arguing that as a 'disease', hepatitis C cannot be taken as an object possessing stable meanings and attributes, but rather, is what Karen Barad might call a phenomenon, always already enacted, the 'meaning' and materiality of which emerges in 'intra-action' with other phenomena. As we have suggested, the ontology of hepatitis C is politics. The thing we know as 'hepatitis C' is a thoroughly political object. Mol's observations can also be extended to subjects. The ontology of subjects is thoroughly political, and those subjects are emergent in action. In this chapter we ask: if we take hepatitis C as a thoroughly political object, what do we make of efforts to treat the virus? How, in short, might we conceptualise the relationship between subject, treatment and politics?

The politics of the overview

The starting point for our analysis in this chapter is the distinction that Mol and Law (2002) draw between overviews, on the one hand, and lists, walks and cases, on the other. We briefly considered some of these distinctions in our introductory chapter, but will revisit each of these below. Overviews are of interest to Mol and Law because, in their view, they are one of the ways in which order is achieved and chaos and complexity are expelled. They write: 'A proper order comes with the illusion that all relations can be qualified and that it is possible to gain an all-inclusive overview' of the phenomenon in question (2002: 14). Overviews come in many forms, including, for instance, classificatory systems of the animal kingdom. Overviews are characterised by closure rather than openness, and by their efforts to 'tame' chaos and complexity – usually through asserting an 'order' and implying a completeness to events, processes or things. Overviews assume that reality follows an identifiable order and, as part of reality themselves, present themselves as orderly in their putative completeness. Against these assumptions about order, Mol and Law express a preference for other epistemological figures, namely lists, cases and walks. They explain that in 'contrast with the overview of the classificatory system ... *lists* are nonsystematic, alert, sensitising but open to surprise' (2002: 16). The aim of lists, cases and walks is, as we noted in the introduction, to produce 'modes of relating that allow the simple to coexist with the complex, of aligning elements without necessarily turning them into a comprehensive system or a complete overview' (2002: 16).

Overviews, as we shall see in this chapter, have an especially significant place in the world of hepatitis C treatment. For instance, many accounts of hepatitis C treatment – in health promotion literature, news media, medical literature, and elsewhere – are readily classed as 'overviews'. They are characterised, that is, by the production of order and the expulsion of complexity, and by the shutting down of possibilities that things might be otherwise. In this sense, overviews are related to another key concept that is central to the analysis we undertake in this chapter – this involves the relationship between 'the centre' and 'the periphery'. According to Bruno Latour (1987) we must always attend to how, in accounts of any 'thing', event or phenomenon, some come to be classified as 'centre' and others as 'periphery'; this is because the arrangement of certain objects/ subjects as central or peripheral works to produce its own ordered account of the world. The importance of the relation between centre and periphery is perhaps best illustrated through a well-known example. Nicolaus Copernicus, Renaissance mathematician and astronomer, is the figure widely credited as the first to propose a heliocentric cosmology (Kuhn 1957; Blumenberg 1987). This heliocentric cosmology posited that, contrary to previous understandings, the Earth was not a fixed, stable object in the cosmos, around which other objects (most notably the sun) revolved. Controversially, he claimed, it was the Earth and other planets that revolved around the sun. Copernicus' re-imagining of the relation between the planets and the sun, while radical at first, gradually came to be accepted as the single and authoritative account of cosmological process. We can say two things about this. First, insofar as the Copernican revolution produced a movement from centre to periphery and from periphery to centre, it produced a shift in scientific logic or 'understanding' of the cosmos. Secondly, and more importantly, it was a thoroughly political event, with implications for how we understand ourselves and our place within the universe. By decentring the Earth and the planets, and moving them – and us, as the Earth's inhabitants – to the periphery, the human itself was subtly decentred.

Let us bring together these two lines of thought – centre/periphery, on the one hand and overviews/lists on the other – to consider the ways they are interconnected. In particular, one of the main methods through which notions of centre and periphery are produced is through the production of overviews; and in this respect, overviews, like notions of centre and of periphery, are thoroughly political. Lists are also political in that, although they can be hierarchical in some cases, they have the potential – depending on their content – to *disrupt* notions of centre and periphery, to destabilise conventional ways of thinking and knowing, and to allow for the element of surprise. This chapter is centrally concerned with questions of centre and periphery in hepatitis C treatment and thus – by extension – the ethics and politics of treatment. In what follows, we consider what counts as centre and what counts as periphery in accounts of hepatitis C treatment, how these distinctions are performed/achieved, why these distinctions are important and, finally, why it is that such divisions might be problematic. The chapter is not simply an attempt to document each of these things; it is also an exercise in challenging conventional accounts of centre and periphery in narratives about hepatitis C treatment. In this respect we aim to produce an account of hepatitis C treatment – but not an overview. The chapter will conclude with a non-hierarchical and non-ordered list of features we identify as associated with treatment. The purpose of this is to resist the temptation to reduce chaos and complexity, or to suggest that the analysis in this chapter is comprehensive. These are issues to which we will return. In the meantime, we begin by looking at the treatment overview.

An overview of treatment

Our analysis begins with two short overviews. The first overview appears in the
Australian Government's *National Hepatitis C Strategy 2005-2008* (Department
of Health and Ageing 2005), and reads as follows:

> With an estimated 16,000 new infections each year, the demand for treatment
> is likely to increase substantially. The efficacy of treatment is improving and
> it is now possible to cure hepatitis C completely in around half of the people
> being treated. Cure not only improves quality of life for those who successfully
> undergo treatment, but also reduces the risk of passing the virus on to others.

For our purposes, the most striking feature of this first overview is the way
in which it provides an account of what hepatitis C treatment 'does': it cures
around half of the people who undergo it, improves quality of life and has
broader public health benefits, insofar as it reduces the risk of new infections.
The second example is taken from a document released by the Hepatitis C
Support Project in 2008. Entitled *A Guide to Hepatitis C Treatment Side Effect
Management*, the document is directed towards people contemplating treatment.
It lists a number of reasons why the reader might consider trying therapy to cure
– or 'clear' – the virus. Although this example takes the form of a list (insofar
as it includes a series of dot points) it bears all the hallmarks of a conventional
overview. This is because it works to produce an ordered account of treatment
(through an explanation of the things that treatment 'does') and specifies
relations (between medicine and its subjects; and between subjects and their
friends/family/others). It also expels complexities – both in the decision-making
processes associated with treatment, and in the experience of treatment itself.
As it does so, it presents itself as complete. What precisely is excluded and why
these exclusions are significant will become clearer as this chapter progresses.
Reasons to contemplate treatment are:

- To improve your health;
- To live longer;
- To feel that you have done all that you can do;
- To be alive for your children, grandchildren, and loved ones;
- To experience life and all it has to offer;
- To simply get rid of the virus;
- To put hepatitis C and its treatment behind you;
- To have children;
- To reduce symptoms and increase your quality of life;
- To prevent liver cirrhosis and liver cancer;
- To help you reach personal and professional goals;
- To avoid being a burden to others.

In the same text, readers contemplating treatment are encouraged to adopt a 'positive attitude' and to cultivate and express gratitude for 'the opportunity to take this treatment' (2008: 2). Implicit, then, is a recognition that treatment for hepatitis C is onerous, and that those contemplating it may need to be convinced of the merits of doing so. Taken together, these two overviews imply at least three sets of ideas, each of which bears on the other:

1. First, we can identify ideas about hepatitis C as disease. The overviews imply that hepatitis C produces negative health effects, as well as a reduced life expectancy. This much is conveyed through the claim that treatment will improve overall health (therein assuming that all people with hepatitis C experience a health deficit) and that treatment will help people to 'live longer';
2. Secondly, we can identify ideas about the subject living with hepatitis C. Here, the suggestion that one might undergo treatment in order '[t]o feel that you have done all that you can do' instantiates the idea that responsible citizens make an effort to improve their health (here, to undergo treatment), or that good health is achieved through action on the part of the subject (so that even if a cure does not eventuate, the subject might experience some form of improvement);
3. Thirdly, and most importantly, the overviews reproduce a set of understandings about medicine, and about the relationship between medicine, disease and the subject. In both, medical care appears as a privilege or 'opportunity', and as capable of producing personal, interpersonal, professional and spiritual transformations. Medicine, in this sense, figures as both 'heroic' and transformative', and as an agent of mastery. As noted in Chapter 1, these figures are also common in medical accounts of developments in knowledge and practice for hepatitis C. For example, McHutchison and Fried described their review of recent developments in treatment as a summary of results of 'clinical trials of these agents that have set *new standards of care* for treating chronic hepatitis C' (2003: 149, our emphasis). These depictions of hepatitis C medicine as 'heroic', 'positively transformative' and 'masterful' must be read alongside the rather more sobering aspects of hepatitis C treatment in action. We will revisit these briefly before proceeding with the chapter's main line of enquiry.

Hepatitis C treatment

Every year around 3,000 people commence treatment for hepatitis C infection in Australia (Hopwood 2009). In other countries, such as the United States, the picture is less clear; a recent study by Volk, Tocco, Saini and Lok (2009) found that treatment rates were declining. At present, medical treatment for hepatitis C takes the form of 'combination therapy'. This involves two drugs: pegylated interferon and ribavirin. People take both substances for either 24 or 48 weeks, the length of treatment for any individual depending upon a range of factors, including genotype (Hopwood and Treloar 2007). The aim of treatment is known as 'sustained virological response', or SVR, as Hopwood and Treloar (2007: 250) explain:

> An SVR is attained when a polymerase chain reaction test (a process which amplifies pieces of the genetic make-up of a cell or virus to detect its presence) at six months post-completion of treatment reveals an undetectable viral load for HCV. In such instances, one is deemed to be cured of HCV infection.

According to Körner (2010: 273), 'treatment success is between 50 and 80 per cent'. Rates of 'clearance' vary according to the age, gender, severity of disease and genotype of the patient (McHutchison and Fried 2003). A high proportion of people discontinue treatment before the completion of their 24 or 48 week period (Hopwood and Treloar 2007). As we have already mentioned, treatment for hepatitis C is recognised to be onerous. This is not only because of the length of commitment required but because it can involve a range of potentially severe and unpredictable side effects. These side effects include lethargy, nausea, alopecia (hair loss), myalgia (muscle pain), flu-like symptoms, inability to concentrate, fluctuations in mood, changes in libido, depression, anxiety, weight loss, anorexia, suicidal ideation, paranoia, anaemia, diarrhoea, vomiting, skin rash, insomnia, leukopemia (reduced white blood count), stroke, irritability and cough (Hunt et al. 1997, Dieperink et al. 2000, Kraus et al. 2000, Fried 2002, Dieperink et al. 2003, Keating and Curran 2003, Hopwood and Treloar 2005, Raison et al. 2005, Yu et al. 2006, Zickmund et al. 2006, Majer et al. 2008, Körner 2010). Although this remains in dispute, there is also the possibility that some of these side effects will be permanent.

Analogies are sometimes drawn between combination therapy and chemotherapy for cancer, perhaps in an attempt to acknowledge the severity of treatment for some people and the challenges it can produce. Whilst the comparison is useful as an explanatory device, we must also be cautious in making it. This is because, most obviously, chemotherapy is not delivered in the politically charged environment of injecting drug use and drug addiction. Nor do the recipients of chemotherapy figure as sources of horror, disgust and shame, in the same ways as do people living with hepatitis C. This is significant, as we shall argue, for understanding hepatitis C treatment as phenomenon, and for grasping its politics, ethics and 'effects'.

In Australia, as in other Western liberal countries, the uptake of treatment is ethically complex and politically charged. One of the main subjects of contention relates to levels of uptake. In short, the claim made by some is that uptake levels are too low and need to be increased. In 2006, for example, the Ministerial Advisory Committee on AIDS, Sexual Health and Hepatitis, Hepatitis C Sub-Committee, called for rates of treatment to be trebled (see Treloar and Rhodes 2009). One reason offered for increasing rates of treatment is 'to prevent the expected increases in people with advanced liver disease' (New South Wales Health 2008: 23) and the associated 'burden' on the health care system in future years. Additionally, some have called for treatment uptake to be increased because of its preventative potential, insofar as a surge in 'clearance' rates will have a likely (although not proven) downward effect on new transmissions into the future (Vickerman, Miners and Williams 2008). As the first author (Suzanne Fraser) has argued elsewhere (Fraser and Moore, 2011), calls for the increased uptake of treatment represent a conflation of individual benefits and rights with public health benefits and objectives. This is just one reason why we might want to approach the push for increases in uptake of treatment with some caution.

As we noted at the outset, however, there are a range of other reasons why we might be cautious about the enthusiasm that hepatitis C treatment can sometimes provoke. Before any major public health push for increases in treatment is embraced there are many more questions we need asked. Why, for instance, push for increases in the number of people undergoing treatment for hepatitis C infection when it is widely recognised to be onerous and uncertain? Rates of success remain extremely variable, depending upon genotype, and patients face the prospect of multiple, serious and ongoing side effects. A common response to questions about success rates for hepatitis C treatment is to refer to its increasing 'effectiveness'. Given the side effects and negative after effects listed above, as well as the difficulties attendant upon predicting a positive outcome, the question of what constitutes 'effectiveness' must be asked. How, that is, do we define success, or effectiveness, if treatment itself brings a range of harms? The notion of hepatitis C treatment as itself capable of producing harms is especially ironic given the environment within which much treatment is delivered. As we argued in Chapter 4, the vast majority of people living with hepatitis C inject drugs, and it is among this cohort that most new infections arise (Hellard et al. 2009). But injecting drug use is commonly understood as an inherently risky, dangerous and harmful activity. In light of this, how might we conceptualise the 'harms' associated with hepatitis C, injecting drug use and drug 'addiction' if harms are also associated with the main form of medical treatment available? What counts as 'harmful' in this context? How and why are some phenomena constituted as 'harmful', 'safe', less harmful' or 'more harmful' than others? Why are some risks legitimate and others not?

And there are yet other questions. If, as we have already argued, the hepatitis C positive subject figures – literally and symbolically – as a source of horror and disgust, how might we conceptualise treatment if one of its stated aims is to clear the virus from the body of the subject, and in so doing, cure her or him? What, in short, does hepatitis C treatment seek to cure? What does treatment *treat*? We can draw together the various concerns articulated in the previous section in a single question that guides the approach in this chapter: 'What does hepatitis C treatment do?' If, as we have been arguing throughout this book, hepatitis C must be understood as a thoroughly political object, so in turn, must treatment. In taking this approach in the rest of the chapter, we will again draw on Mol's observation that ontology and reality are political, iterative and multiple. We also take up ideas from feminist, queer, race and cultural theorists on the constitution of subjecthood. Finally, using these theoretical tools, we will explore the ways in which treatment reproduces a kind of 'binary logic' *vis-à-vis* addiction and drug use. The next section considers these various theoretical perspectives and their utility for a critical analysis of hepatitis C treatment.

More than one and less than many

In recent years the Enlightenment understanding of the subject as unified, self-contained and anterior to social relations has been thoroughly critiqued by scholars in fields as diverse as feminist theory, queer theory and postcolonial studies. Here, we draw on the work of two theorists, one based in feminist/queer theory and the other in postcolonial studies, both of whom theorise the body and subjectivity in ways that can contribute to our understandings of hepatitis C, treatment and the subject. We begin with a now famous statement from feminist and queer theorist Judith Butler on the 'domain of the abject'. The first author has previously considered the utility of this work for injecting drug use (Moore and Fraser 2006) and it is worth revisiting for present purposes. As Butler (1993: 3) explains in the seminal feminist text *Bodies that matter*:

> This exclusionary matrix by which subjects are formed thus requires the simultaneous production of a domain of abject beings, those who are not yet subjects, but who form the constitutive outside to the domain of the subject. The abject designates here precisely those 'unlivable' and 'uninhabitable' zones of social life which are nevertheless densely populated by those who do not enjoy the status of the subject, but whose living under the sign of the 'unlivable' is required to circumscribe the domain of the subject.

According to Butler (1993: 3), the domain of the abject emerges as the site 'against which – and by virtue of which – the domain of the subject will circumscribe its own claim to autonomy and to life'. In the same passage, she continues:

> In this sense, then, the subject is constituted through the force of exclusion and abjection, one which produces a constitutive outside to the subject, an abjected outside, which is, after all, 'inside' the subject as its own founding repudiation.

For Butler, the subject surfaces through a process (or through processes) of exclusion and inclusion, so that the materialisation of bodies/subjects depends on the simultaneous production of their (imagined, presumed, enacted) antitheses: the body/domain of the 'abject'. The abject is a 'site of dreaded identification' for the subject, thus the abject exists in counterpoise to the subject, against whom it is produced through the forces of exclusion.

Another theorist who has written extensively on the production of subjects is the French philosopher Michel Foucault. Although Foucault's work is wide-ranging and diverse, he is probably best known for his theorisation of power. In order to understand the salience of Foucault's work on power we must first say a few words about traditional (or 'orthodox') models of power, as it is these that Foucault set out to challenge. According to Foucault, the orthodox perspective of power is one in which it is understood as an entity 'held' by a few and imposed upon or directed at a (larger, oppressed) category of others. This theorisation of power manifests most obviously in Marxist work on relations of capital, where power is envisaged as vested exclusively (or primarily) in the means of production, or in the 'State apparatus' (Foucault 1980a: 59-60). In the field of health and medicine, this approach to power is most closely associated with the 'orthodox' medicalisation thesis (Lupton 1997). This perspective sees the medical system as an 'institution of social control' (Zola 1972) and doctors as the agents of social control. According to this approach, social control is effected and perfected through the application of expert medical knowledge onto 'bodies'/'patients'. This approach is underpinned by an orthodox version of power because it assumes that doctors 'hold' power and impose it on patients; in this sense, the orthodox medicalisation thesis emphasises the passive and powerless nature of patients relative to medical professionals (Bury 1997; Armstrong 1984). In both the orthodox medicalisation thesis, and in Marxist analyses of capital, then, power is conceived as *imposed*, from the top down, *by* the powerful few, *upon* the vulnerable many.

As we noted in Chapter 4, such an approach to power is problematic. First, it is unrealistic and unsustainable, to the extent that it positions both 'doctors' and 'patients' as uniform and homogeneous collectivities. It also implies that doctors alone are agentive, and that patients are incapable of acting on the world in any way. This is an especially troubling position for marginalised groups (such as people living with hepatitis C and people who inject drugs), because, as marginalised and stigmatised populations, they are already understood to be lacking in agency, irrational and lacking enterprise. By extension, this model of power treats attempts to transform the lives of the marginalised and stigmatised as destined to fail because it offers little hope that they can act upon the world. In so doing, it offers little hope that things can – and might – be otherwise.[1] A different way of understanding power is therefore required not only for theoretical reasons, but as a political and ethical imperative. It is here that Foucault's work on power becomes most useful.

------

1   Of course, Foucault has not escaped such criticisms himself. Feminist theorists have been especially vocal (see, for example, Hartsock 1990). As Lois McNay (1991: 125) has pointed out, insofar as Foucault suggests that power is 'everywhere', he implies that agency and resistance might not be possible; she argues that this renders his work of limited use to feminists, because Foucault's 'lack of a rounded theory of subjectivity or agency conflicts with a fundamental aim of the feminist project to rediscover and re-evaluate the experiences of women'.

Challenging this orthodox approach to power, Foucault argues that traditionally dominant sovereign forms of power had now given way to disciplinary forms of power. In a famous statement on the need for a radical re–conceptualisation of power, Foucault called for philosophers to metaphorically 'cut off the King's head' (Foucault 1984: 63) and look instead towards the multiple and infinitesimal formations and functions of power. In this sense, Foucault urged a shift in conceptual focus as well as practice, suggesting that 'nothing will be changed if the mechanisms of power that function outside, below and alongside the State apparatuses, on a much more minute and everyday level, are not also changed' (Foucault 1980a: 60). The central point of contention for Foucault is that power is not a 'localised phenomenon', existing only in the hands of certain groups, such as doctors (1980a: 59-60). Instead, power is – in his words – 'everywhere' (1978: 93). Power is exercised via a multitude of 'infinitesimal mechanisms' (Foucault 1980b: 99) including the 'clinical gaze' through which bodies are classified as abnormal, treated and normalised (Foucault 1977/1995: 184). It is also exercised in other ways, including via self-discipline. Power operates *through* individuals, including doctors, patients, self–help groups, friends and family (Foucault 1980c: 142). In Nancy Fraser's (1981: 279) view, Foucault's theory of power is best understood as:

> capillary. It does not emanate from some central source, but circulates throughout the entire social body down even to the tiniest and apparently most trivial extremities.

For the reasons we have already discussed, this reconceptualisation of power is especially resonant for the study of health, illness and medicine.

For the purposes of the argument we make in this chapter, there is one further, crucial element of Foucault's theorisation of power to consider. To the extent that Foucault challenges ideas of power as applied from the 'top down', he also challenges the notion of power as always and inherently repressive. In the Foucauldian medical model, power is not necessarily a repressive phenomenon; indeed, power can be a *productive* force (Foucault 1984: 60-61). Power can, in Foucauldian terms, actually make things, objects and subjects. At the heart of Foucault's theory of power is the concept that power is not necessarily 'prohibitive' but that it is also 'productive' – of knowledge and of selves (Foucault 1980a: 59-60; 1984: 60-61). For example, rather than seeing medical encounters as solely repressing women (as many feminists have argued they do) we can see them as constituting women in particular ways – as 'healthy', 'pregnant', 'fertile', 'infertile', 'old', 'young', 'fit', and so on. Here, subject positions are produced in and through medicine, but these are not necessarily or automatically 'repressive'. This aspect of Foucault's work on power (which sees it as productive, as opposed to repressive) has been criticised as politically and ethically neutral (see Fraser 1981; Taylor 1984).[2] However, Foucault's distinction

---

2 According to Nancy Fraser, Foucault calls 'too many different sorts of things power and simply leaves it at that' in circumstances where 'it is essential to Foucault's own project

between the productive and repressive dimensions of power does not necessarily mean that power is never repressive; similarly, taking power to be 'productive' should not be mistaken for seeing it as necessarily 'positive'. Indeed, the distinctions between 'fertile' and 'infertile' bodies, or between 'healthy' and 'unhealthy' citizens regularly works to marginalise and stigmatise those so constituted. Moreover, these constitutions are often historically and culturally specific, developed out of medical 'knowledge' and practice (Foucault 1973). Most important here is the recognition that subjects are produced through power, to investigate how this takes place, and to analyse the political implications of these processes.

How might the work of Butler and Foucault be mobilised in an analysis of hepatitis C treatment? Most significantly, both theorists reject conventional understandings of subjects as foundational, or anterior to social relations. In Butler's case, it is the taken-for-granted essentialist reading of the prior (sexed/ gendered) body/subject that demands challenge. Women, as we know, have been historically disadvantaged by accounts of the social world that attribute too much influence and agency to matter. Butler's concern is thus to challenge determinist accounts of reality (as in, for instance, the body) through which matter comes to count for *everything*, via a turn to the relation between discourse and matter. In Foucault's case, the concern is with the ways in which power, as everywhere and infinitesimal, operates to produce subjects, and objects. Although the work of these theorists has many differences, they share a view of the subject as emergent in action, as surfacing, enacted or performed, through practice (although see Barad 2003, on the limitations of Butler's approach). The crucial point here is that the production of subjects is a political and ethical practice with implications for relations of power. The processes through which individuals, groups and collectivities emerge are often obscured, however; taken as 'natural', as given, in the order of things. The point is thus to shine a light on these processes and in so doing, make visible the assumptions we hold about what difference *is*, how difference *emerges*, and the processes through which difference is made.[3]

---

that he be able to distinguish better from worse sorts of practices and forms of constraint' (1981: 286). Charles Taylor has argued that Foucault's position with regards power is, in essence, neutral (Taylor 1984: 156). The second author has considered these debates in her work on endometriosis (Seear 2009a). For more, see Hoy (1986), Patton (1989), O'Malley et al. (1997) and Stenson (1998).

3   In earlier work (Seear, Fraser and Lenton, 2010), we have previously considered some of the ways in which subjects might otherwise surface through practices of articulation. This work involved a consideration of the work of race and cultural studies theorist Sara Ahmed (2004a, 2004b) on the articulation of emotions. In that work, we examine the role emotions articulated in relation to hepatitis C *work* to surface bodies, delineate them and produce collectivities. In that paper, we argued that the articulation of sympathy needs to be read not simply as an expression of individual feeling, but as a material-discursive, political and ethical practice that operates to surface bodies and collectivities. The articulation of sympathy towards some people living with hepatitis C and not others works to materialise two distinct collectivities: the first being those people who have acquired hepatitis C

In the work we have just described, Butler and Foucault are concerned with disrupting the binaries of subject/object, or discourse/materiality. The operation of binaries is a subject of special significance to the field of illicit drug use, because people who inject drugs are often constituted through a binary logic. In accounts of drug use and addiction, the following binary pairs are frequently encountered: voluntarity/compulsivity, autonomous/dependent, active/passive, reason/emotion, strong/weak, masculine/feminine, order/chaos, control/lack of control and authentic/false. In each pairing, drug use, addiction and people who use drugs figure as symbolically aligned with the second (and devalued) of the pair. People who inject drugs are thus considered to be dependent, compulsive, passive, emotional, weak, feminine, chaotic, lacking control and inauthentic (Fraser and valentine 2008). The binary logic of drug use/addiction leads us to a consideration of the final body of work that is relevant to this chapter – work on the constitution of addiction. According to Eve Sedgwick (1993), the notion of 'addiction' produces and enforces an opposition between voluntarity and compulsion (see also Valverde 1998; Moore and Fraser 2006; Seddon 2007; Fraser and valentine 2008; Seear and Fraser 2010). In Sedgwick's view, the disease model of addiction produces and reproduces a binary logic which positions voluntarity and compulsivity as absolute opposites. Central to the notion of addiction is a fantasy of voluntarity. As Sedgwick (1993: 134) explains:

> The scouring work of addiction attribution is propelled by the same imperative; its exacerbated perceptual acuteness in detecting the compulsion behind everyday voluntarity is driven, ever more blindly, by its own compulsion to isolate some new, receding but absolutised space of *pure* voluntarity.

In the same way that the notion of compulsivity is produced through reference to its imagined opposite (voluntarity) so are the dualisms we have listed above. Accordingly, the dualisms of addiction, such as chaos and order, autonomy and dependency, authenticity and falsity, are a fiction.

As we have noted in previous chapters, the 'proper' subject of late modernity is closely associated with the first feature in each of these dualisms. This 'proper' subject, as we know, figures as autonomous, responsible, rational, enterprising and choosing. In contrast, 'addicts' are generally understood to be dependent, irresponsible, irrational subjects, who make 'disordered' (Seddon 2007) choices and lack free will (see Fraser and valentine 2008; Moore and Fraser 2006). Accordingly, people who use drugs, and drug 'addicts', figure as less-than-full citizens in late modern, Western, liberal contexts. So how do these ideas bear

iatrogenically, and who are the recipients of sympathy, and the second being those who have acquired hepatitis C in other ways (most notably injecting drug use) and who are, presumably, undeserving of sympathy. Some of the implications of the articulation of emotion are examined elsewhere in this book.

on the question of treatment for people living with hepatitis C? As we have already noted, people living with hepatitis C are constituted as symbolically and literally synonymous with injecting drug use and drug addiction. To this extent, it becomes tempting to leap to a conclusion in which people living with hepatitis C emerge as less-than-full-citizens. This presumption requires a more thoroughgoing analysis, however. Assuming as we do that the subject is not anterior to treatment, and that the subject positions of citizen and non-citizen are performed, enacted or materialised in action, it becomes possible to argue that subjects are made in treatment. But what kinds of subjects does hepatitis C treatment enact? And how, moreover are they enacted? The remainder of the chapter is concerned with these questions, with the relationship between treatment, subjectivity and citizenship. In what follows we consider three enactments of the subject (and medicine) through accounts of treatment. In keeping with previous chapters and our use of Mol and Law's ideas, we argue that hepatitis C treatment produces more than one subject position, but less than many. In this, treatment both challenges and reproduces stereotypical understandings of 'people who inject drugs'. By and large, however, treatment produces people living with hepatitis C as unstable, chaotic, irrational, failed subjects. This positioning occurs first, through pathways into treatment for hepatitis C and secondly, through the experience of treatment itself. It is of enormous political and ethical significance, as we shall see, because it reproduces them as less-than-full citizens, and impacts directly on the lives of those so constituted.

Order and chaos

As we noted earlier, people who use drugs are frequently characterised through 'a taxonomy of two polarised conditions, the negative state of "chaos" and the positive state of "order" in the form of stability' (Fraser and Moore 2008: 740-41). According to the authors, this chaos/order binary serves to delegitimise drug use and people who use drugs through their symbolic association with the devalued subject position of 'chaos'. But what does chaos actually mean? According to Fraser and Moore (2008) the notion that people who inject drugs are always already 'chaotic' is commonplace in drug policy, practice and popular culture, but closer examination of the field demonstrates that notions of chaos and order are both 'poorly defined' and 'poorly elaborated'. The meanings given to stability, chaos and order are not themselves stable, fixed, or self-evident. They are performed in action. Such performativity in the domain of treatment, we suggest, materialises some bodies as chaotic and others as ordered.

The first way in which notions of chaos and order emerge in action is through injunctions from medical professionals to people about the conditions of treatment. One participant, Ellen (female, 58 years) had not been through

treatment herself. She had, however, been associated with many people who
had undergone treatment, observing:

> At the liver clinic that we were involved with, the clinicians spent some time
> deciding on what their approach to illicit drug use would be, and they put in
> place these, what appeared to me pretty arbitrary, sort of benchmarks. And
> their advice to clients was, and these were people wanting and going through
> treatment, not to inject more than two or three times a week. And in fact that
> was one of the major issues with clients [...] it doesn't matter how a doctor
> says something like that to a client, the clients will hear that as clinically
> driven [...] that's what the majority of clients concluded. That, so if they
> didn't adhere to this advice, then therefore their chances of a good outcome
> would be diminished. [There] was nothing clinical about it, it was entirely to
> do with stability.

In this extract, Ellen describes her observations of hepatitis C treatment. As
do Fraser and Moore (2008), she touches upon the notion that 'instability'
is arbitrary, poorly defined and emergent in action. In this specific instance,
'stability' figures as euphemism for reduced drug consumption. Reduced drug
consumption thus comes to figure as a precursor to treatment in circumstances
where there is no evidence that injecting drug use bears any relationship to
treatment success. Although reduced drug consumption is claimed to have a
strictly medical role – that is, that it will enhance the prospect of treatment
success (see Hellard et al. 2009) – injunctions to limit drug use have more
specific aims, such as reducing chances of re-infection as a result of fewer
injecting episodes. It is also closely associated with assumptions about treatment
compliance – namely, that people will present for appointments and adhere to
the treatment regimen if they are taking fewer illicit drugs.

Notions of 'stability' and 'instability' also emerge in the ways pathways
to treatment perform chaos and order. People living with hepatitis C regularly
report being encouraged to take up treatment by counsellors, general
practitioners, peer educators and others. As we noted briefly in the previous
chapter, a common theme to emerge from interviews with participants is their
subjection to a set of expectations about the necessary preconditions to a course
of hepatitis C treatment. One participant, Stuart (male, 39 years) explains
he was keen to have treatment, but three separate attempts to access it were
unsuccessful. On the first occasion, he says:

> I went to [an inner city health service] and I inquired about [treatment] and
> the nurse said 'where are you living and what are you doing?' She said 'well
> our policy is to not give hepatitis C therapy to anybody that's not in stable
> accommodation', because it's very expensive and people who aren't in stable
> accommodation, they're likely not to see the whole treatment through and

that sort of stuff, that's what was explained to me. So I was told to come back and apply for it once I'd gotten myself sorted out.

In his second and third attempts to access treatment, Stuart was reportedly again deemed ineligible by his health care professionals. In the following extract, he explains his own understanding of why he was not eligible:

> But around about the age of 37, I was listening to the radio and they were talking about a hep C trial for a pill, not for injections, but actually trialling a pill of this therapy ... I went there and, well the reason why I was in hospital in the first place was because I had a suicide attempt, and that's ... I told them this at the [hospital] and they said 'sorry we can't put you into our study'. I thought 'oh yeah, great, oh well'. I can't remember what they said to me, but they said 'oh, you can't go for this study', but then I heard there was hepatitis C at [another hospital], there was hepatitis C treatment available at [another hospital]. So I've gone there, and I've gone there and told them I had hepatitis C and would I be able to have the therapy. I didn't tell them about the suicide attempt because I wanted to try the therapy. I actually went to my local GP, who's been my GP, and still is, for quite some time, and told him that I was going to the [hospital] and I was going to get the hepatitis C therapy. And he said 'yeah, fine' and applied for and got the [disability] pension, because I was expecting to get the therapy. And about the third time I went there, a doctor came out and said 'oh, we've got it on your records that you've had a suicide attempt, we can't give you the therapy'.

Stuart is performed as chaotic and disordered (in his vulnerability) in his interactions with health care professionals. Here, the meaning of stability is reproduced through these interpersonal negotiations; it is not anterior to these social relations, but, rather, materialises as part of them: as part of the negotiations between Stuart and his doctors. Incidents from Stuart's past and present coalesce with other factors to become instances of instability. These factors include Stuart's subject position as a 'person who injects drugs' and as 'a person living with hepatitis C', his interest in pursuing treatment in a context where others act as gatekeepers to that treatment, the revelation of his housing status and the exposure of his prior suicide attempt (first, through his own admission and then later, through hospital records of the event). It is also important to acknowledge here that we cannot take Stuart's account of his doctors' behaviours as evidence of reality, only evidence of Stuart's reality. In any event, a past history of mental health issues is often cited as a contraindication for hepatitis C treatment. Accordingly, the act of excluding participants from treatment on mental health grounds functions – even when well-intentioned – as an explicit acknowledgment of the harmful or risky potential of hepatitis C treatment.

Until now we have been arguing that notions of instability emerge in and through the clinical encounter. The point here is that instability and stability are produced through relations, and are not anterior to them. Crucially, however, these processes of emergence and production actually co-exist alongside and resonate with, other discourses which similarly position injecting drug use and people who inject drugs as unstable and chaotic. Indeed, as several authors have pointed out, drug use is widely assumed to be 'unstable' and 'chaotic', and in accounts of drug use and the lives of people who use drugs, regularly constituted as such (Keane 2002; Fraser and Moore 2008; Fraser and valentine 2008). What this means, then, is that the notion of 'instability' is reproduced – but not *remade*, in the sense of being challenged, distorted, or radically reoriented – in accounts of the pathway into treatment. Moreover, notions of instability are – in some instances – also reproduced (although again not remade) in the pathways into treatment itself. In Stuart's account of his treatment, then, instability is enacted through a process of convergence, where lack of 'stable' housing arrangements and (past) mental health problems come together and are performed as a form of (his) instability. Stuart's current housing arrangements and past history of mental health issues are reconstituted as evidence of his 'instability' and 'chaotic' lifestyle, and, by extension, his lack of fit with hepatitis C treatment. Most importantly, Stuart's subject position as 'chaotic' and 'unstable' emerges through these articulations. He is not, that is, 'naturally', 'essentially' or 'inherently' unstable, but enacted this way through dual articulations that suggest that lack of continuity in housing is evidence of instability, as is a prior suicide attempt. This is then the first example of how hepatitis C treatment enacts its subjects: through processes of articulation in the pathway to treatment, it can perform it subjects as chaotic, disordered and unstable. As we shall see, this has potentially devastating consequences for people who inject drugs, as well as policy responses to drug use, addiction and hepatitis C, and for the lived experience of hepatitis C. Most obviously, it ensures Stuart foregoes the possibility of occupying a new, less stigmatised subject position: that of someone without hepatitis C.

The dominant attribute in the binary pair of order and chaos is 'order', or 'stability' (a term that is, like its opposite term instability, poorly defined, unbounded and constituted in action). Some of our participants describe emerging as 'stable' subjects through their efforts to adopt certain recommended practices prior to the start of treatment. As Karl (male, 41 years) explains:

> Well I couldn't really see that I could do anything about hep C until I was prepared to actually become healthy, you know. So that means stop using drugs, stop using alcohol, later I stopped cigarettes, and then I started to sort of change my diet. So as I'm doing that, then I sort of prepared myself and of course the latest thing I'm doing is being on the treatment. So, and hopefully this will clear it and then that will be the past.

Here, Karl emerges as a compliant and 'orderly' subject through his enactment of a set of activities in preparation for treatment. These include becoming 'healthy', abstaining from illicit drug use and alcohol consumption, quitting smoking and changing his diet. Like 'chaos', notions of 'order' (most obviously, abstinence from drug use) are reproduced through Karl's pathway into treatment. In this way, as Karl takes steps to change his life, improve his diet and reduce his consumption of drugs, his actions come to both reflect and reproduce 'order'. Like Stuart, Karl believes that there is an expectation that he perform a particular version of subjectivity (responsible, stable, orderly) as a precondition to starting treatment, but the particular constellation of 'orderly' behaviours is enacted through reference to an imagined sense of what order might look like. Karl is thus enacting a form of subjecthood he understands is required to gain access to treatment and in so doing, reproducing that very same 'order'.

This understanding – that one needs to get one's life 'in order' as a prerequisite to treatment – was widespread in the data. In another interview, Long (male, 34 years) describes his understanding of the preconditions for treatment:

> You have to be off the drug for a while, you have to be a certain criteria. I'm not sure about that but I know you have to be off drugs for a certain amount of – year – and you have to put your name down for a while. And interferon is very, what's it, radioactive or whatever, it's really toxic, something like that. Actually, I do know somebody that had interferon. Apparently he can't sleep with his partner while he had the interferon. And every time he go to the toilet or something he had to flush twice. Something, it's very contaminated stuff so, yeah, I'm not really looking forward to that test, I'd rather wait for something better.

In this extract, Long restates the common understanding that abstinence from injecting drug use is a prerequisite for treatment. He expresses far less enthusiasm for treatment than does Karl, primarily because of the 'toxic' effects he fears will follow. Crucially, even if Long chooses not to take up treatment, treatment performs him. This is thus another example of the productive and constitutive effects of medicine: the production of subjects as chaotic or disordered, and the difficulty of enacting subjecthood outside this binary logic. So here we have additional ways in which treatment enacts its subjects: pathways in to treatment perform them as ordered and stable (when subjects 'comply') and as disordered when they do not.

Unlike Stuart, Karl appears to have the material resources to support his enactment of 'ordered' subjecthood. This is a key point, because it alludes to the mutual relationship between subjectivity and neo-liberalism. What we mean by this is that the subject positions 'orderly' and 'chaotic' rely upon material-discursive arrangements (access to rehabilitation services, or to psychological support, or to financial resources) that are not available to everyone. As such, the enactment of both the 'chaotic' and 'disordered' subject positions bear some relationship to the 'proper' subject of contemporary, Western, liberal discursive contexts we outlined earlier. We will recall that the 'proper' subject of late modernity figures as autonomous, responsible, rational, enterprising and choosing and in this sense is expected to be able to perform proper subjectivity through self-reliance. As Lisa Blackman (2006: 209) among others, has explained, this notion of autonomous selfhood is a 'fiction'. As has been widely argued, material constraints operate to reduce individual capacity for autonomous action and enterprise (Seear 2009a; Daykin and Naidoo 1995). In this way, as Nikolas Rose (1999: xxiv) argued in some of his earlier, more critical work, we need to acknowledge that the claims to autonomy and individuality associated with autonomous selfhood can be 'if not illusory, then imaginary'.[4]

Read together, Stuart and Karl's accounts reveal that pathways to treatment work to forcibly constitute some subjects as ordered and others as chaotic. In a related sense, notions of 'order' and 'chaos' are made through mutual processes of enactment and counter-reference (Fraser and Moore 2008). Both 'chaos' and 'order' are produced and reproduced through processes of distancing in which particular practices emerge as the domain of either the 'subject', or the 'abject' (Butler 1993: 3). The first conclusion we can therefore draw about hepatitis C treatment is that it can produce drug use and people who use drugs as chaotic and disordered. What we mean by this is that treatment can enact people living with hepatitis C as either (or both) orderly or chaotic. Most often, however, they are enacted as chaotic. Crucially, the aim and the function of treatment is to produce them as ordered. In this respect, hepatitis C treatment produces 'order' as the 'proper' subject position of contemporary Western liberalism, but obscures the ways in which order is itself an invention, insofar as order actually depends upon the 'fiction' of autonomous selfhood.

Success and failure

As Catherine Waldby (1996: 1) argues in the opening of her book *AIDS and the Body Politic*, 'Declarations of epidemic are declarations of war'. In that work, Waldby explores the relation between HIV/AIDS and the body politic. An extension of these insights to hepatitis C as 'war' seems apt, for the language of 'battle' and the imagery of 'war' figure regularly in popular and medical accounts of the virus. Writing for *Bloomberg Businessweek*, John Carey (2006) depicts scientists as 'waging war on hepatitis C' and deploys military metaphors to account for this battle of wills.[5] The virus, he suggests, has an 'ability to hide from the body's defences'. He goes on:

> Like most viruses, the hepatitis-C bug commandeers the host's cellular machinery to make copies of itself ... Think of the immune system as having a built-in burglar alarm. Cells roam the body equipped with little detectors, or receptors, on their surface. These receptors seek out and attach to foreign

---

4   In his work on responsibilisation, Graham Burchell (1996: 24) agrees, pointing out that the autonomous subject is 'not so much a given of human nature as a consciously contrived style of conduct'.

5   Available   at: http://www.businessweek.com/technology/content/feb2006/ tc20060221_196821.htm

invaders, such as viruses. Once the receptor finds such an invader, it sends out an alarm, mobilising the immune system to attack the invader ... In the case of the hepatitis-C virus, the cells successfully identify them as foreign invaders. But the alarm signal they try to send doesn't get through ... So even though the 'burglar' is detected, the alarm never gets sent to the immune system's police station.

In Carey's account, these functions of the virus are enacted as 'mysteries' that have been 'unlocked' by the heroes of science. Medicine and virus are locked in battle, waging war. Later, Carey writes that treatment figures as the great 'hope' of people living with hepatitis C. Treatment emerges as the alternative to war, the means, that is, by which war will be brought to an end. But this account of the relationship between treatment, subject and war is very much at odds with accounts of treatment in our interviews. For many, treatment is a kind of war itself. But what exactly is the object of that war? What are the spoils over which the war is being fought? And who are the antagonists?

In our participants' accounts of treatment, the subject, medicine and virus are literally and symbolically produced as in battle with one another. For some, such as Barbara (female, 52 years), this battle begins before treatment starts:

> **Barbara**: No, no, I was going to clear. I, actually I did a really weird thing, but to mentally prepare myself I was, I was a warrior and I shaved my head.
>
> **Interviewer:** (Both laugh) fantastic.
>
> **Barbara:** Oh my God. Not bald, but very short and I was going, I was there ready, take it on, take it on. And a friend of mine said 'oh, I like your hair'. How they could say that? It looked disgusting, but mentally I had prepared for this battle, but unfortunately I lost. I never, I didn't respond. So that took a while to get over.

In spite of Barbara's determination to beat her bug, treatment was not successful. Another of our participants, Hillary (female, 54 years) explains her sense of despair when she learned that the virus had not been cleared through treatment:

> When I failed treatment I think it was – I started – I had – I felt quite devastated and felt like I had nothing, and really no one to talk about it to.

Importantly, both Barbara and Hillary produce an account of treatment failure in which they figure as central. If we pay careful attention to the language both women use, we see that Barbara positions herself as the loser in a mental and physical war waged against her virus, expressed through phrases such as 'I was a warrior', in 'this battle', 'but ... I lost', 'I didn't respond'. Similarly, Hillary explains that 'I failed treatment' (not that treatment failed her), and later, adopting terminology in frequent use in the hepatitis C literature, referred to herself as a 'non-responder'. In both accounts, agency is attributed to the knowing subject, and in so doing, functions to produce the subject as deficient, as source of failure.

It is not enough to end our analysis of success and failure in treatment at this point because, as Law (2004: 83) reminds us, 'what is being made present always depends on what is also being made absent'. What is made absent in these accounts of treatment failure? If these accounts enact subjects as sources of failure, then they simultaneously enact medicine as passive in the face of deficiency, not as source of failure, but as antithesis to it. As we noted in Chapter 1, medical literature produces treatment as success in spite of the persistence of the virus, because the virus' persistence is attributed to the treated subject. Medicine thus emerges as heroic in two ways: first, through its war against the virus, and second, through its war against the subject, who materialises as an obstacle to medicine's unfettered heroic potential. Of course these moves – from centre to periphery, and back again – are not stable in space and time. Just as developments in treatment for hepatitis C shift – or to borrow the language of Mol and Law (2002) – slop, churn and swell in space and time, so do medicine, virus and subject materialise differently. We cannot, to paraphrase Mol and Law (2002), pin medicine down, nor can we pin down the subject. But we can locate particular versions of medicine's agency, its status as 'centre' or 'periphery', in accounts of its action. Where discursive constructions of medicine in public health and medical literature constitute it as heroic and patients as a possible source of failure, it is not surprising to find these ideas emerging in the self-understanding of patients too. It is patients, ultimately, who pay the price for these configurations, through enrolment into a broader discourse which positions them as moral and personal failures, and through their symbolic and literal positioning, as sources of horror, disgust and shame as people who inject drugs. In these ways the price of treatment and its discursive constitution is high, yielding enormous personal, political, ethical and material costs. Still more effects will become visible in the future, if as John Carey (2006) and many others often say, a cure for hepatitis C is just 'around the corner'. What this means, at the very least, is that new treatment regimens are on the horizon, with new effects for the subject. There is every chance things will get better, but just as much reason to approach revolutions in medicine with skepticism.

In any case, the accounts of treatment offered by our study participants function to produce medicine and its subjects in ways that appear (at first glance) to challenge conventional understandings of agency and the dualisms associated with each (medicine as order/active, subject as chaos/passive). Instead, just as medical literature performs the subject as failure and medicine as success (Chapter 1), so too does treatment. One of the most important observations we should make at this point in our analysis is that it is not just Barbara and Hillary who speak of treatment failure in this way. Indeed, those working in the field of hepatitis C will immediately recognise the kind of language both women use because they mobilise terms widely used in the sector in practice. From our own experience as researchers in the hepatitis C field, attending forums and seminars, presenting papers and listening to papers at conferences, reading medical, health promotion and self-help literature, and speaking with health care professionals, peer educators and other experts, it is common to hear some or all of the following expressions *vis-à-vis* the subject in treatment:

- The subject is non-compliant;
- The subject has failed treatment;
- The subject is a non-responder;
- The subject has discontinued treatment;
- The subject is unstable prior to treatment;
- The subject requires stability in order to undertake treatment;
- The subject is vulnerable in treatment;
- The subject is liable to fail to complete treatment;
- The subject requires encouragement to remain in treatment;
- The subject has failed to respond to treatment.

In each instance, the subject is positioned at the centre of accounts of treatment. It is, for example, the *subject* who fails treatment (rather than treatment failing the subject), the *subject* who discontinues treatment, the *subject* who fails to comply with or adhere to treatment, the *subject* who is unstable, the *subject* who discontinues treatment and the *subject* who fails to respond. As our analysis in this chapter demonstrates, however, subjects do not exist prior to the treatment that performs them. All of these subject positions (and others not mentioned here) can therefore be said to be enacted through, or materialised via the combination pegylated interferon and ribavirin treatment they are seen to choose, and the concepts, instruments, personnel and activities that help to make it.

Treatment as despair

Thus far this chapter has addressed two main dimensions of treatment: its relation to order and chaos, and to success and failure. The final theme this chapter addresses is that of treatment side effects. Common side effects of treatment were listed earlier. In our interviews, most of these, and some others, were described. These descriptions resonate with the narratives of recovery from treatment collected by Max Hopwood and documented in *Recovery from Hepatitis C Treatments* (2009). In that report, Hopwood (2009: 12-13) noted that participants had problems:

> [i]n attributing the cause of ongoing physical and psychological health problems after treatment; were they an outcome of the treatment drugs, difficulty adjusting to finishing treatment, underlying liver damage, or in those people who did not clear their infection, the return of hepatitis C? Or were their health problems a mix of all or some of these possible causes, and if so, how much was attributable to each one?

In this chapter we are also concerned with the complexities people face in identifying the cause of new or continuing health problems after treatment, but in what follows we pursue a different line of inquiry. It begins with a story of 'existential' despair told to us by one of our participants.

For at least one interviewee, Giuseppe (male, 41 years old), treatment for hepatitis C was a momentous experience of 'existential' significance. A sustained period of combination therapy left Giuseppe feeling, in his own words, 'confused', 'really confused' and 'angry'. In the following extended passage, Giuseppe explains his first day on treatment:

> I suppose [my doctors] did what they could. They informed me of all the side effects. And, I was aware of the stigma attached, I mean, I was a user anyway, I was a squatter, you know what I mean, so there was stigma attached to even just existing at the time, before that. So, you know what really freaked me out, is that they let you go home with that pegylated interferon [... and my peer support worker] said to us, you know, 'four hours after you have that injection' – this is where I felt I was let down by [my clinic] the most – was they didn't tell me how heavy that was going to be like. He goes 'four hours, and if you don't feel nothing you might be one of those lucky people that has no side effects'. I thought fuck, and I remember walking down the stairs at home, and I was saying to [girlfriend], I was saying 'I might be one of those freaky fucks that is going to get away with, this is going to have no effect'. I remember twenty minutes later I started getting cold, within an hour, I couldn't control how much I was shaking. She wanted to ring an ambulance. I didn't want her to ring an ambulance, because, you know, I thought I was being a real pussy about it. But I couldn't control how much, it was like having a dirty hit. When you have, when people inject, if there's a little bit of, speck of dirt in the spoon and the filter doesn't stop it from going up and it goes into your bloodstream, it overrides all the dope and you, it's like a toxic reaction. You start vomiting and getting really cold. It was like that. And I thought, fuck, what are they doing? Why isn't this in a [hospital] in-patient sort of situation? Why have they let me go home and do this? I was really freaking out. He said, you know, 'take one Panadol' or something ... It was like I said, it was like I was having a toxic, like I was in toxic shock.

Later in the interview, Giuseppe explained that this pattern continued for a further six to eight weeks. In that time, Giuseppe's white blood cell count 'plummeted', his lips bled, and he lost around ten kilograms. Unable to hold down food, he vomited often, became depressed and suicidal. For Giuseppe, hepatitis C treatment was transformative. It left him feeling, at times, that 'the rest of the world is crazy and I'm the only sane one'. As he explained:

> Well I used to ask my treating doctor, or the psychologist or whatever, where does the interferon stop and I begin? Like how much is this affecting what I'm

thinking, how much of what I'm thinking about is me, and how much is it the interferon affecting me?

Treatment produced in him a kind of 'existential crisis' and – to return to the metaphors of war discussed earlier – a battle for survival:

> ... so the treatment, the interferon sort of accentuates, it makes it more profound, my existence is being put in peril. Or [it creates the sense that I have] put my existence into peril. Just as the virus wants to survive, so did I. I wanted to survive just as much as the stinking fucking virus.

Here, Giuseppe articulates a sense of confusion about who he *becomes* through treatment. This sense of confusion about the self, subjectivity and place in the world, is common to the treatment experience. Karl (male, 41 years) speaking of his own experience of a range of side effects following treatment, described those symptoms as:

> ... fairly general. That's fairly general, you know. I had other, it's difficult with hepatitis C in a way, because there's so many potential side effects that *it's sometimes hard to know what is hepatitis C and what is something completely different*, you know?

In a similar sense Hillary (female, 54 years) reported depression during her treatment regimen, but was confused about the 'source' of these feelings, saying 'Whether it was related to my hep C or not I don't know'. The sense of confusion about what becomes of the subject in treatment, through treatment, as summed up in Giuseppe's existential question ('where does the interferon stop and I begin?') illustrates in a new way the point, made throughout this chapter, that subjects are produced, transformed, performed and enacted in treatment. In addition, Giuseppe's articulation of existential despair works, like other forms of emotional articulation (for a discussion of this area, see Ahmed 2004) to destabilise assumptions about the prior (drug using) subject who is 'unstable', 'chaotic' and 'inauthentic' and about medicine as always productive of subjects who are 'ordered', 'stable' and 'authentic'. Also, and of considerable significance for present purposes, Giuseppe's articulation of existential despair challenges the way 'risk' is typically mobilised in accounts of both illicit drug use and medicine. Most obviously, his account of treatment disrupts the conventional distinction between illicit drug use as always and inherently 'risky', (a form of dangerous consumption) and of medicine as non-risky, or inherently safe (a point we touched on in the previous chapter). Of course, observations about the riskiness of medicine are not new, having populated sociological literature in the study of health and medicine over several decades. One example can be found in the work of Ivan Illich (1976) whose early critique of medicine produced an influential account of its iatrogenic potential. But questions of medicine's safety, value and efficacy take on special significance and added urgency in the context of hepatitis C and injecting drug use, especially for the purposes of health education policy and practice. In the face of Giuseppe's sense of existential peril, how should we respond to the tensions, contradictions and challenges that treatment throws up? How do we approach this, as a practice, that strives to reduce harms, on the one hand, but, in so doing, may actually produce them? This is a matter to which we will return shortly.

What else might we take from these accounts of treatment as inducing despair? As Helen Keane (2002) explains in her book *What's Wrong with Addiction?*, addicts are constituted in popular, psychological and scientific discourse as 'inauthentic'. The 'falsity' of the addict is often positioned as a direct effect of their use of 'addictive substances'. Speaking to a passage from a specific text called *Drugfree: A Unique, Positive Approach to Staying Off Alcohol and Other Drugs*, Keane (2002: 75) writes:

> The implication is that the substance is actually bad: it lies to the brain, programs the belief system like a cult leader indoctrinating an innocent follower. Similarly, the authors talk about the effect of drugs on the mind as a form of deception; drugs gain a hold on us by 'clouding our ability to see or to believe that their use is against our own best interests'. By using artificial means to feel artificial pleasure, the addict is already in the realm of untruth, even before any statements are made about his interior being.

Keane describes accounts of the body-drug encounter as thoroughly enmeshed with the dualisms of natural/artificial and true/false, with some relationships (with friends and partners) constructed as 'natural' and others (with alcohol, drugs) as 'artificial'. At the risk of labouring our point, it should by now be clear that such distinctions do not hold. In the context of hepatitis C treatment, this is so for at least two reasons. First, these dualisms rely on the widely critiqued notion that subjects exist prior to their enactment, and secondly, on an account of substances as possessing natural, or inherent properties. This much is conveyed by the notion of 'artificiality' and associated claims that substances such as alcohol and illicit drugs are inherently dangerous or chaos-inducing. Claims that position substances as either and only 'natural' or 'artificial' rely on a version of matter as fixed, stable and non-changeable. Such a notion of matter as stable also reinforces a central polarity in discourses addressing both medicine and drug use: medical substances are performed as always inherently 'good' and illicit substances as always inherently 'bad'.

Revealed in these accounts is the emergence for some people of combination therapy as risky and dangerous; as producing chaos, inauthenticity and disordered subjectivity. This is even more apparent in some accounts which position therapy as analogous to (although not the same as) some illicit drugs. For example, when Hillary (female, 54 years) says: 'I felt like it was absolute chaos, really', she appears to be describing illicit drug use, or the 'drug using lifestyle'. Instead, she is describing an established and publicly funded form of medical treatment. Other participants depict therapy in similar terms, as 'contaminating', 'toxic', or 'alien'. A few expressed reluctance to undergo treatment because they did not wish to ingest 'toxic chemicals'. As Lucinda (female, 39 years; iatrogenically acquired hepatitis C) explains:

> I hate putting chemicals in my body, and that was why, for years, people were always like, 'Oh well [hepatitis C is] a junkie disease' and I mean, my partner, my husband has hep C, and he got it through intravenous drug use, and you know, whatever, however you get it, it doesn't bother me. But it wasn't, and the whole thing was, I really hate chemicals in my body, I really hate it, it freaks me out. So I didn't like the idea of having to go on treatment, and I resented it deeply.

In this extract, combination therapy emerges as a dangerous form of consumption, akin to illicit drug use. These close associations – between combination therapy and illicit drugs – featured regularly in discussions of treatment. Giuseppe, we will recall, described his first dose of hepatitis C treatment as similar to a 'dirty hit'. Others, such as Cuc (female, 29 years) explained a series of side effects that provoked memories of drug detoxification:

> Hair loss, I just couldn't get out of bed on some days, back aches, aches all over, I was depressed, very depressed, just no energy at all. I was, very mild sweats. I hate the sweats, 'cause it just reminds me of, you know, quitting. But it wasn't as bad as detox, but very similar.

Here, Cuc draws parallels between the experience of undergoing treatment for hepatitis C and the experience of quitting drugs, or undergoing detox, thus blurring the lines between illicit drug use as always and inherently harmful and medical treatment as always or inherently healing.

These are not the only lines blurred in treatment. As noted above, Lucinda (female, 39 years) acquired hepatitis C iatrogenically. She explained that treatment performed subjects in ways that blurred the boundaries between her preconceived notions of different people living with hepatitis C. She could no longer distinguish between those who had acquired hepatitis C iatrogenically and those who had acquired it through injecting drug use:

> I used to come to the support group, and I used to look at people, and I was trying to work out, how much of their side effects were just from the treatment and how much were from mismanaged lives, or from drinking or diet, or there's all sorts of other effects. I was always trying to work that out. But [treatment] just didn't seem good.

In this extract, treatment emerges as simultaneously *homogenising*, insofar as it performs subjects as (primarily) chaotic, disordered, unstable, sick, weak and inauthentic, and *multiplying*, enacting additional and new subject positions. But – and this is our key point here – in spite of treatment's simultaneously homogenising and multiplying tendencies, it is most often one, devalued subject position that is produced in action: that of the non-citizen. This is the subject position most often materialised in and made available through pathways into treatment, and in the administration of treatment itself. In this way, combination therapy both disrupts and reproduces a narrow version of subjecthood regularly associated with injecting drug use and addiction. It is this, ultimately, that speaks to the constitutive power of medicine, as politics, and brings into stark relief the contradictions, tensions and challenges at the heart of contemporary medicine. Although there are occasional exceptions (such as medicine's willingness to acknowledge 'mental health' issues as a risk factor in treatment), medicine is generally ill-equipped to address the existential crises it induces. Instead, it 'others' the need to do so, and the role of alternative forms of expertise in so doing.

Conclusion

A consideration of the life and work of Nicolaus Copernicus may seem an odd place to end a chapter on the lived experiences of hepatitis C treatment. But as this chapter has sought to make clear, questions about what counts as 'centre' and what counts as 'periphery' are vital for any consideration of the ethics and politics of hepatitis C treatment. As Latour (1987: 226) explains, 'For a Copernican revolution to take place it does not matter what means are used provided this goal is achieved: a shift in what counts as centre and what counts as periphery'. As is the case with hepatitis C as disease, what counts as centre or periphery is moveable and constantly changing, not given. But how these shifts occur is always and inherently political. One example of this is found in the centrality of medicine to agency at some points in time (when treatment is successful) and its retreat to the periphery at others (when treatment fails – or, more precisely, when 'the subject fails treatment'). In this specific instance, medicine's retreat from centre to periphery is complemented by a mutual appointment (of the subject) to centre. In addition, as we have already noted, these movements, from centre to periphery, or from periphery to centre, and back again, materialise in space and time, and then disappear, alongside shifts in the nature of medical treatment. What this means is that the range of movements that we have identified in this chapter (from centre – periphery – centre) are themselves in a state of constant motion. Indeed, by the time this book appears in print, these constellations might already have vanished, only to be replaced by a new set of movements, swells, travels. Doubtless the arrangement of medicine and its subjects, of centre and periphery, has changed since the introduction of pegylation to interferon, thus increasing rates of clearance for some people.[6] As new treatments emerge, we

---

6 For more information on developments in treatment, and research findings suggesting that the combination of pegylated interferon with ribavirin is a superior form

will witness still more movements in the relation of medicine and its subjects. Crucially, because these movements are inseparable from the ethics and politics of injecting drug use and addiction, however – indeed, *because these movements are politics* – every shift equates to a politicisation of both medicine and the subject. Most often, as we have argued throughout this chapter, these movements figure to the detriment of an already grossly stigmatised and stereotyped population, reproducing them as non-citizens, as horrifying and as shameful.

What this means is that in the same way that hepatitis C treatment is always already in motion, so, too, are the subjects it enacts. In this respect, the account of treatment we have produced in this chapter is both fractional and fleeting; it captures only some of the movements that treatment produces as well as movements that might already have passed. But this is not to say that the account of treatment detailed in this chapter is redundant, or that there is little value in tracking current arrangements. Medicine reproduces these subjects in ways that are *already very familiar to us* – it performs them as 'chaotic' and 'unstable', and reproduces people who inject drugs as 'failed' subjects or 'non-citizens'. Moreover, medicine also produces *itself* in ways familiar to us: as heroic and transformative, and valorises and demands certain subject positions at the same time that it enacts others as less valuable and valid. The outline of treatment we have drawn in this chapter demonstrates some of the ways medicine produces and reproduces subjects in ways that fit neatly with stereotypes of the 'addict'. This has the effect of stigmatising and marginalising the individuals and groups that medicine seeks to 'help'. We would have less to be concerned about if treatment *remade* its subjects anew every time it acted upon them. But, to return to the point we made earlier, medicine *reproduces* subjects, objects and culture as much as it inaugurates them; it rarely *remakes* any of these things anew. Given the push to increase treatment rates we identified at the start of this chapter, critical accounts such as ours are of considerable utility, as is careful scrutiny of the enthusiasm with which treatment is being embraced at the policy level in countries such as Australia.

This analysis has been an exercise in challenging conventional accounts of centre and periphery in narratives about hepatitis C treatment. Like any account of a phenomenon, ours enacts its own version of hepatitis C treatment too, through the choices we have made about the inclusion of some interview extracts to the exclusion of others, the construction of themes and the production of patterns, in the arrangement of materials, and the order (literally and metaphorically) of things. To return to our consideration of lists, cases, walks and overviews at the outset of this chapter, we wish to close in a manner that avoids the usual turn to order and the overview. As Mol and Law (2002) remind us, overviews are themselves performative; they make their own order, and in so doing, seek not only to expel

---

of treatment to its predecessors, see: Manns, McHutchison, Gordon, Rustgi, Shiffman, Reindollar et al. (2001); Fried, Shiffman, Reddy, Smith, Marinos, Goncales et al. (2002) and Hadziyannis, Sette, Morgan, Balan, Diago, Marcellin et al. (2004).

that which is chaotic or complex but to forget what has been expelled, insisting that 'what belongs to them is drawn together and properly assembled'. Moreover, overviews tend towards oversimplification, collapsing complexity (Law and Mol 2002: 7). To be clear, then, our aim in this chapter has not been to produce a more complete overview (in the sense of a definitive account) of hepatitis C treatment. We have sought to instead provoke a critical re-evaluation of things that treatment can do, whilst recognising that treatment will always do more and new things, other things, things not accounted for in these pages.

As we observed at the outset, overviews of treatment are extremely common and tend to arrange medicine and its subjects in particular ways – almost always positioning the former as heroic and transformative and the latter as failed, chaotic and transgressive. Our decision to resist making of this chapter an overview of treatment is an intellectual, ethical and political choice, emerging from a desire to resist collapsing the complexity of treatment. It would not do to simply replace one overview of treatment with another. This choice does not come without risks, however. Indeed, the choice to refrain from producing a hierarchical list of the features of treatment opens up the possibility that the proceeding analysis becomes a merely random set of observations about the things treatment can do, without any claim to these enactments being politically or ethically significant. In this sense, our resistance to the 'overview' speaks to a central tension in the work of Mol and Law – it risks, as with the work of Foucault – a kind of political and ethical neutrality. To be absolutely clear, then, things that happen in treatment – things that treatment does – can have devastating consequences for many. These consequences require investigation and analysis. While it would no doubt be easier to present these analyses as authoritatively complete, we find ourselves bound by a competing concern. Claims to order and authority of this kind are consistently deployed against, and presented as alien to, those individuals and groups this book seeks to understand.

The list with which we close this chapter is intended to inform the deliberative processes that posit treatment for hepatitis C as a vital plank of public health and harm reduction strategies. At the very least our list should provoke a reconsideration of the assumption that treatment is always useful for people living with hepatitis C (although we recognise, of course, its benefits for some). The list is intended to be both non-hierarchical and incomplete. We invite readers to add to it. Indeed, it is destined for nothing other than change:

- Movements between the centre and periphery are always inherently political;
- Notions of centre and periphery bear upon hepatitis C as 'disease' and its subjects;
- Subjects are hived off, demarcated and produced as both 'centre' and 'periphery' in treatment, and these moves are political in their orientation and effects;
- Subjects and objects move from centre to periphery and back again, with

these moves political in their orientation and effects;
- Subjecthood is emergent and multiple;
- As with all subjects, people who use drugs are a very diverse population;
- As do all subjects, people who use drugs enact multiple subject positions;
- The subject positions most frequently performed in treatment are normative;
- One may perform some, all or none of these subject positions at the same time;
- Treatment is politics;
- Treatment is ontology.

Conclusion
The 'Smoldering and Fluctuating Course'

This book has attempted to execute a series of linked paradoxes. Its aim has been an ambitious one: to produce a new account of hepatitis C that is, in itself, of very modest ambition. In it, we have analysed the materialisation of the disease across a range of influential discursive domains, making claims about the effects of the discursive constructions we encounter, questioning their utility and value, seeking to disrupt them and show how they are enfolded into cyclic iterations of stigma and discrimination. At the same time, however, we have taken up the conceptual and methodological challenges posed by our own critique. If those most directly affected by hepatitis C, people who inject drugs, are disadvantaged and marginalised by the complacent liberal idealisation of reason and order, we are obliged to engage with reason and order skeptically ourselves. The book constructs and exercises reason in the analyses each chapter undertakes, and produces a degree or form of order as it does so. Yet it also questions reason and order, asking that we (authors and readers alike) remain alert to all those elements othered in the production of these forms of reason and order.

This is all very well, of course, but alongside our modesty – our wish to lay claim to a partial perspective, partial order only – runs a parallel wish that the observations and critiques generated by this perspective be taken seriously and used in remaking understandings of, and responses to, hepatitis C in new, less constraining and costly ways. Do these simultaneous wishes make a paradox too? Only if the sole basis for according critique attention and legitimacy is a claim to (inevitably mythical) status as objective reason and impartiality. So in this way, this book metaphorises the paradoxical struggle people who inject drugs might be said to face. Intentionally or otherwise, in the pursuit of pleasure, the rejection of simplistic distinctions between natural and artificial sensation, and the refusal of fictions of bodily autonomy and purity, they enact a critique of Western Enlightenment reason and its philosophical and material sequelae. Their actions and practices constitute a challenge to our complacent assumptions about the exclusive value of reason and order. How should we greet this critique? As always already flawed and illegitimate? As a wound or lesion in the social fabric in need of diagnosis and cure? This book, we hope, suggests not. Its aim has been to actively draw upon the critique enacted by injecting drug use to expose the arbitrary and self-serving forms of order generated within authoritative and influential responses to hepatitis C, within, that is, medical, public health and self-help materialisations of disease and those who have it.

Injecting drug use has been, that is, our key conceptual resource. It has laid bare the ethical need to think beyond the rational, the pure and the authentic. In doing so it has demanded we seek innovative conceptual and methodological tools. We have drawn these from scholarship equally skeptical of simplistic claims to reason and order: mainly science and technology studies and feminist science studies. We began by consulting Bruno Latour, whose disquiet about certain interpretations of fact inspired him to distinguish between 'matters of fact' and 'matters of concern'. It is the latter notion, he argues, which best describes knowledge and being. Indeed, this book has been nothing but an attempt to materialise hepatitis C as a matter of concern. Seen as a 'thing' constituted in action, a site of dealing and dispute in its ontology, hepatitis C emerges as always already political force, always already enacting subjects and their possibilities, always already enacted by these too. Hepatitis C is not a myth or a nightmare, yet it is not simply a fact or an object either. It is a material-discursive process and resource through which worlds are made. As Susan Leigh Star observes, 'power is about whose metaphor brings worlds together' (1991: 52). As we have seen, hepatitis C is both metaphor and matter, its metaphorical manifestations shaped by the politics of drugs, injecting and disease.

In seeing hepatitis C as a matter of concern we have drawn on a range of other theoretical tools. We have thought disease in terms of lists, cases and walks, we have recognised knowledge-making as mess-making, as crafting and gathering, as the reiteration and creation of presence, absence and otherness. Perhaps most consistently (or iteratively) we have understood hepatitis C as more than one and less than many. Without this understanding of disease as ontologically multiple and open to change, the purpose of our critique would be far more limited than it has been. By identifying the self-serving and limiting aspects of knowledge about and responses to hepatitis C, we dare to expect that these can change, and therefore, that the materiality of hepatitis C and its effects can change, be re-made, reiterated in new ways. This is at the centre of our paradox of modesty alluded to earlier. Although we acknowledge the partiality of our critique, we also expect, and feel obliged, to produce insights and recommendations for change, albeit tinged with caution about claims to academic objectivity, comprehensiveness and conclusiveness. It is a delicate line to walk – a 'smoldering and fluctuating course' (Martell et al., 1992: 3226) – that, if we fancy to learn from hepatitis C's apparent success, allows adaptation and resilience even as it must relinquish identity and essence and therefore some authority.

What has the book's smoldering and fluctuating course led us to conclude? Here there are many areas to cover, some limited to this disease in particular, and some to disease and its ontics more broadly. Three main (interrelated) threads of inquiry can be identified in the foregoing discussion, although there are many more, no doubt, or at least many others more obvious to differently primed eyes. These threads are:

1. The ways in which matters of concern, in our case the disease hepatitis C, must be 'held together';

2. The mutually constitutive relationship between knower and object of knowledge and the dynamics by which the integrity of the former may be preserved in the particular framing of the latter;
3. The role of othering and all its costs and rewards in constituting matters of concern as matters of fact.

Regarding our first point, it is perhaps clear by now that this book has taken as its core task the demonstration of at least some of the ways hepatitis C is held together. Using examples and illustrations from medical journal articles, health promotion materials, self-help books and the words of people diagnosed with the disease, the chapters have explored precisely how a vague and disparate collection of symptoms, risks and prospects are made into a coherent disease, entailing, despite the instability of its core attributes, a stable and predictable – if undesirable – set of social and political effects. We have also tracked, as we will explain in more detail below, how this set of effects is in part constituted from the work done to preserve the epistemological credibility of the discursive agents we examine, in particular, medicine and public health. Thus, for example, the uncertainties of symptomatology are attributed to the slipperiness of the virus rather than to the limits of scientific knowledge, and the uncertainties of treatment to the unreliability of patients rather than to the limits of medical expertise. Does the epistemological preservation of one phenomenon always necessitate the undermining of another? We hope not but it appears that, at least through these examples and in this case, in the shifting of agency and responsibility we have identified, the two are dynamically linked.

In Chapter 1 we began with what we called a 'quasispecies epistemology' – a set of observations about the constitution of phenomena drawn figuratively from hepatitis C's own genetic multiplicity. This epistemology made the following observations about the making of phenomena:

1. Their ontology is constant motion;
2. They are made in repetition. This always entails error, and creates change;
3. Error and chaos are productive – they are enfolded in, rather than antithetical to, order;
4. They are always already more than one and less than many;
5. Causation in this making is multidirectional and non-linear; and
6. Sameness and difference in and among phenomena are contingent.

These observations attempted to capture the routinely obscured features and processes by which phenomena are made to hold together. Hepatitis C changes constantly across time and space in knowledge. It develops as a social object, as a phenomenon, through the almost constant re-production of error – of partial and even subsequently discredited knowledge about it. The disorder or chaos entailed in this error does not disrupt the apparently orderly production of hepatitis C as a coherent object. Instead it founds it and is the condition of its possibility. At the same time that the object is made over and over as singular and coherent, it is also made over and over as multiple. A range of discursive strategies operate to manage this multiplicity, to discipline it as merely the substance of singularity. The meaning and materiality of hepatitis C make each other. The two are ontologically and epistemologically inseparable, although the discursive strategies holding hepatitis C together tend to represent the relationship unidirectionally, with materiality taken to be the cause of meaning. The relationships between hepatitis C and other phenomena, such as HIV – that is, their sameness and difference – are constantly in motion, contingent upon political forces and not given in nature.

These are complex processes by no means easy to pin down. Yet identifying them and introducing the skeptical reflex they demand into the centre of liberal Enlightenment epistemology is, finally, our goal. To quote Jacalyn Duffin once more (2005: 32), 'diseases are not immutable objects lying around waiting to be unearthed like potsherds in an archaeological dig'. In Chapter 3 we revisited this concept, showing how hepatitis C is remade in self-help discourse through discussions of HIV, emotions and iatrogenesis. Of course, Duffin's observations apply not only to disease but to all phenomena, including those taken, sometimes all too conveniently, to be thoroughly understood. What is injecting drug use? What is infection? What is responsibility? What, as Rose might ask in the context of new biological knowledges and practices, is a citizen, and how does one qualify as one? Each and every phenomenon animating our discussion is made and remade in the politics of hepatitis C. Each and every one might be otherwise.

Regarding our second point, the book has illuminated an important set of relations between knower, be this science or more particularly medicine in this case, and object of knowledge. In Chapter 1, we demonstrated the mutually constitutive nature of knowledge about disease and notions of scientific progress. We critiqued the way in which preserving the epistemological integrity and authority of the latter has at times entailed the enactment of particular, sometimes pejorative or unjustifiable, discursive formulations of the former, such as those constituting patients as failures. In Chapter 4, we tracked this tendency into public health understandings of individual engagement with knowledge about hepatitis C. These understandings tend, we argued, to construct people who inject drugs diagnosed with hepatitis C as incompetent or negligent if they do not continually maintain their knowledge of medical developments in the area. In turn they tend to present the goals of public health, however inattentive they may be to the material and social constraints faced by their target populations, as self-evidently reasonable and productive. Instead, we argued, based on the interviews we conducted, inattentiveness to the (smoldering and fluctuating) course of medical knowledge about hepatitis C, the changing advice about prevention and the changing opportunities offered by treatment, is just as reasonable and productive as attentiveness. Further, we recommended that proponents of public health responses subject the field itself to the questions about responsibility and agency so often aimed only at affected individuals.

In keeping with these observations about the dynamics operating between knower and object of knowledge in this field we also noted, in Chapter 2, the need to reconsider the ways in which the hepatitis C virus is figured in health promotion. We suggested a move away from accounts of the virus as duplicitous, unpredictable and cunning, and recommended that health promotion openly acknowledge the limits and partiality of medical knowledge about the virus. We also recommended that variations in symptomatology be represented less a function of the virus' unpredictability and more as a reflection of medicine's limited capacity in grappling with these variations. In this way, we argued, more credible and potentially less stigmatising discussions of the disease would be produced. In our view, health promotion should not be conceived as beholden to the authorisation processes attached to science and medicine. There is no doubt it should consider medical knowledge about health and disease a key resource, but this, it seems to us, all too readily entails an expectation that this knowledge be presented as conclusive and comprehensive. Not only is this inaccurate, it is also unconvincing to readers. As such it erodes trust and hampers effectiveness.

This last matter relates also to our third point – the need to remain alert to what is othered in the making and holding together of hepatitis C. As we argued in Chapter 1, the way in which testing is discussed in the medical literature is very instructive. Notions of mystery and silence are mobilised to present the virus as lurking in the body, eluding detection. The disease, in this formulation, is silent yet active. Noting this, we argued that characterising hepatitis C in this way positions scientific endeavour as transparently seeking knowledge – as actively and neutrally and comprehensively listening for signals which, when properly detected and decoded, will solve the 'problems' of disease. Following Law and Mol's comments about silence, however, we observed that this presentation of 'silence' as an attribute of the virus leaves scientific practice unquestioned. Is the virus silent, or are we just not listening in the right way?

This last question exemplifies a further aim of the book – the examination of relations of centre and periphery as they constitute hepatitis C, and the experimental reversal of these relations to illuminate disease ontics in new ways. Thus, in Chapter 4 we concluded that in understanding individual engagement with treatment, there is a need to question the continual search for new ways of accounting for or changing individual decisions and actions. Instead, we would do well to reverse centre and periphery, placing the circumstances, priorities and perspectives of prospective patients at the centre of our logic, and the assumptions and demands of medicine at the periphery. This reversal would allow us to see better the limits of those measures offered by medicine, and the constraints operating on individuals in their pursuit of biological citizenship. We argued that shifting the focus in this way generates new questions beyond the familiar ones that assume we need to make people who inject drugs better, more resourceful, biological citizens. Why even aspire to reverse the direction of our questions in this way? Because questions about drug using subjects are asked repeatedly, while questions about the biopolitical circumstances and forces through which they are constituted are asked relatively rarely. Are expectations about people who inject drugs *themselves* rational, responsible and reflexively constituted, or do they make unreasonable assumptions about agency, responsibility and the place of medicine? In that agency and responsibility are key attributes of the citizen in contemporary liberal democracies, these questions carry a great deal of weight in thinking through citizenship processes. This book has attempted to spell out how the mutual constitution of disease and subject also opens up and closes off particular avenues for citizenship.

Perhaps most pressingly, we conducted our reversal so we could ask a further question, one about paradox. What happens, we asked, when hepatitis C-positive people who inject drugs are seen both as flawed, addicted subjects for whom rationality and self-management are but fantasies, and as reasoning health consumers in possession of the resources and ambition to choose onerous health measures as an expression of their agency and efficacy? Again, what should we make of these measures themselves? How 'rational' and 'reasonable' are *they*? *Who* precisely, to recap the questions we raised in Chapter 4, acts on faith, compelled by expectations and desires, hopes and fears? We argued that medicine, public health and their exponents operate beyond the realms of the rational no less than do those they wish to re-make as rational biological citizens.

Chapter 5 undertook a reversal of a similar kind, scrutinising the dynamics of centre and periphery in asking how hepatitis C treatment acts upon and performs subjects. We argued that questions about what counts as 'centre' and what counts as 'periphery' are vital for any consideration of the ethics and politics of hepatitis C treatment, and that centre and periphery shift in response to the changing politics of disease. We took as a key example of this the way in which medicine is located at the centre of agency at some points (when treatment is successful) but retreats to the periphery of agency at others (when treatment fails – or, as is most commonly said, when 'the patient fails treatment'). Here, these shifts from centre to periphery produce important political effects. Glory, it seems, belongs to medicine, failure and disappointment to the (already failing, already disappointing) hepatitis C patient/'drug addict'.

This state of affairs, as with the others we have illuminated and queried in this book, is not given in nature, instead it is materialised in practice. It is ontics and as such, could be otherwise. Let us return once more to the questions posed by Mol which were first quoted in the Introduction:

1. Where are the options?
2. What is at stake?
3. Are there really options?
4. How should we choose?

Here we have located some of the options for materialising the phenomenon of hepatitis C, discussed what is at stake in its specific materialisations and in the latency of other materialisations, considered the possibility of change and at least some of the actions and measures required to allow change, and made claims about the choices to be made. In doing so we have, to reiterate this too, treated our subject as a matter of concern composed of partial yet not insignificant facts. We have, as was also foreshadowed in the introduction, treated this disease as a 'gathering'. We have gathered it here according to our own ontological and epistemological commitments and perspectives. We have treated it as one of Heidegger's 'things': material object and site of dealing and dispute at once. As Latour (2004: 237) explains in his attempt to walk his own chosen smoldering and fluctuating epistemological course, 'Things that gather cannot be thrown at you like objects'. This book's final aim is to simply (though it is, of course, no simple matter) convert hepatitis C from 'object' to 'thing', from matter of fact to matter of concern, to introduce, that is, the notion that hepatitis C is always already more than one and less than many. It is gathered and regathered in material-discursive practices of all kinds; public health, medical treatment, research and daily life. A gathering, we think Latour is trying to say, can never be a missile. It cannot be used to threaten or harm as it only falls apart in flight. We hope the insights offered here help demonstrate that hepatitis C too falls apart in flight, that it cannot serve as the immutable, self-evident origin of threatening or harmful assumptions and effects that produce stigma, pathologisation, responsibilisation and the rest. If we are still in any doubt as to the merits of disrupting the objectification of hepatitis C as a matter of fact, we need only return to the words of those diagnosed with the disease. Speaking of the burden of hepatitis C, and of the challenge of disclosing his viral status to others, Giuseppe musters this defiant speech: 'Oh, guess what, I've got hepatitis C, judge me if you like, but I'm a carrier'. We dare say things that gather can no more be 'carried' than they can be thrown. Nor can they form the basis for the moral judgments Giuseppe has learned to anticipate and ought to manage.

While the observations we have made in this book emerge from the particular material-discursive domain of hepatitis C, they are also worth thinking through beyond this context, in relation to other diseases and other matters of concern more broadly. Indeed, the three threads we have drawn from our analysis, with which we conclude our walk through the matters of hepatitis C, might also be identified elsewhere:

- All phenomena must be 'held together'. This holding together is always political and demands scrutiny;
- All practices of knowledge production mutually constitute knower and object of knowledge. This dynamic process can locate culpability, silence and failure inappropriately or unjustly; and
- All knowledge is made up of presence, absence and otherness. The costs and rewards associated with particular processes of othering also require scrutiny.

All three threads offer ways into many objects of analysis, but only for those willing to forego the authority, order and conclusiveness promised by conventional epistemology. Indeed, in reversing centre and periphery as we have done throughout this book, in rejecting the overview, and critiquing fantasies of conclusiveness, in proceeding, that is, with due modesty, we have left ourselves no clear way to conclude, no final claim to order and no ultimate flourish of authority. If we consult Law on endings, he is just as likely to say, 'I don't know', and then to turn to metaphor (2004: 156). He seeks, he says, metaphors for the 'stutter and the stop', for 'quiet and more generous' conceptions of knowledge-making. Here, even as we dare to look for and invoke change, we too must necessarily 'stutter' and come to 'stop'. Here, as we embrace modesty as well as the desire to persuade and therefore help to transform, we call for quiet and more generous understandings of disease.

Bibliography

Ahmed, S. 2004a. Collective feelings, or the impressions left by others. *Theory, Culture & Society*, 21(2), 25-42.

Ahmed, S. 2004b. *The Cultural Politics of Emotion*. Edinburgh: Edinburgh University Press.

Alter, H.J. 1991. Descartes before the horse: I clone, therefore I am: The hepatitis C virus in current perspective. *Annals of Internal Medicine*, 115(8), 644-9.

Altman, D. 1986. *AIDS and the New Puritanism*. Sydney: Pluto Press.

Anti-Discrimination Board of NSW. 2001. *C-change: Report of the Enquiry into Hepatitis C Related Discrimination*. Sydney: Anti-Discrimination Board of NSW.

Appelbaum, D. 1995. *The Stop*. Albany, NY: SUNY Press.

Ariss, R. 1997. *Against Death: The Practice of Living with AIDS*. Amsterdam: Gordon and Breach.

Armstrong, D. 1984. The patient's view. *Social Science and Medicine*, 18, 737-44.

Aronowitz, R. 1998. *Making Sense of Illness: Science, Society and Disease*. Cambridge: Cambridge University Press.

Australian Gastroenterology Institute. 1991. *Hepatitis C: An Information Leaflet for Patients and Interested Members of the General Public*. Sydney: AGI.

Australian Injecting and Illicit Drug Users League. 2009. *Inside Out*. ACT: AIVL.

Ballard, K. and Elston, M.A. 2005. Medicalisation: A multidimensional concept. *Social Theory & Health*, 3, 228-41.

Barad, K. 1998. Getting real: Technoscientific practices and the materialization of reality. *Differences: A Journal of Feminist Cultural Studies*, 10(2), 87-128.

Barad, K. 2001. Re(con)figuring space, time, and matter, in *Feminist Locations: Global and Local, Theory and Practice*, edited by M. Dekoven. New Brunswick, NJ and London: Rutgers University Press, 75-109.

Barad, K. 2003. Posthumanist performativity: Toward an understanding of how matter comes to matter. *Signs: Journal of Women in Culture and Society*, 28(3), 801-31.

Barad, K. 2007. *Meeting the Universe Halfway: Quantum Physics and the Entanglement of Matter and Meaning*, Durham, NC: Duke University Press.

Bhandari, B.N. and Wright, T.L. 1995. Hepatitis C: An overview. *Annual Review of Medicine*, 46, 309-17.

Blackman, L. 2006. Inventing the psychological: Lifestyle magazines and the fiction of autonomous self, in *Media and Cultural Theory*, edited by J. Curran and D. Morley. London: Routledge, 209-32.

Bland, J.M. and Altman, D.G. 1996. Measurement error. *British Medical Journal.* 21: 313(7059), 744.

Blumenberg, H. 1987. *The Genesis of the Copernican World.* Cambridge, MA: MIT Press.

Bonkovsky, H.L. and Mehta, S. 2001. Hepatitis C: A review and update. *Disease-a-Month*, 47(12), 610-64.

Bourdieu, P. 1986. The forms of capital, translated by R. Nice, in *Handbook for Theory and Research for the Sociology of Education* edited by J.G. Richardson. New York: Greenword Press, 241-58.

Bowen, D. and Walker, C. 2005. The origin of quasispecies: Cause or consequence of chronic hepatitis C viral infection? *Journal of Hepatology*, 42, 408-17.

Brook, H. and Stringer, R. 2005. Users, using, used: A beginner's guide to deconstructing drugs discourse. *International Journal of Drug Policy*, 16(5), 316-25.

Brownscombe, J. 2004. The uppers and downers of medicalising addiction. *studentBMJ*, 12, 89-132.

Bruce, C. and Montanarelli, L. 2007. *Hepatitis C: The First Year*, 2nd edition. New York: Marlowe & Company.

Brunsdon, C. 1987. Feminism and soap opera, in *Out of Focus*, edited by K. Davies, J. Dickey and T. Stratford. London: The Women's Press, 147-50.

Bunton, R. 1992. More than a woolly jumper: Health promotion as social regulation. *Critical Public Health*, 3(2), 4-11.

Bunton, R. and Burrows, R. 1995. Consumption and health in the 'epidemiological' clinic of late modern medicine, in *The Sociology of Health Promotion: Critical Analyses of Consumption, Lifestyle and Risk*, edited by R. Bunton, S. Nettleton and R. Burrows. London: Routledge, 206-22.

Bunton, R., Nettleton, S. and Burrows, R. 1995 (eds). *The Sociology of Health Promotion: Critical Analyses of Consumption, Lifestyle and Risk.* London: Routledge.

Burchell, G. 1996. Liberal government and techniques of the self, in *Foucault and Political Reason: Liberalism, Neo-liberalism and Rationalities of Government*, edited by A. Barry, T. Osborne and N. Rose. Chicago: University of Chicago Press, 19-36.

Bury, M. 1997. *Health and Illness in a Changing Society.* London: Routledge.

Butler, J. 1990. *Gender Trouble: Feminism and the Subversion of Identity.* New York and London: Routledge.

Butler, J. 1993. *Bodies that Matter: On the Discursive Limits of Sex.* New York and London: Routledge.

Butt, G. 2008. Stigma in the context of hepatitis C: Concept analysis. *Journal of Advanced Nursing*, 62(6), 712-24.

Carey, J. 2006. Waging war on hepatitis C. *Bloomberg Businessweek* [Online, 21 February]. Available at: http://www.businessweek.com/technology/content/feb2006/tc20060221_196821.htm [accessed: 7 August 2010].

Carey, W.D. and Patel, G. 1992. Viral hepatitis in the 1990s, part III: Hepatitis C, hepatitis E, and other viruses (review). *Cleveland Journal of Medicine*, 595-601.

Castel, R. 1991. From dangerousness to risk, in *The Foucault Effect: Studies in Governmentality*, edited by G. Burchell, C. Gordon and P. Miller. Chicago: University of Chicago Press, 281-97.

Cherry, S. 2008. The ontology of a self-help book: A paradox of its own existence. *Social Semiotics*, 18(3), 337-48.

Cichocki, M. 2009. *Living with HIV: A Patient's Guide*. Jefferson, NC: McFarland & Co.

Cohen, M.R., Gish, R.G. and Doner, K. 2007. *The Hepatitis C Help Book: A Groundbreaking Treatment Program Combining Western and Eastern Medicine for Maximum Wellness and Healing*. New York: St. Martin's Press.

Colquhoun, S.D. 1996. Hepatitis C: A clinical update. *Archives of Surgery*, 131, 18-23.

Commonwealth of Australia Department of Health and Ageing. 2005. *National Hepatitis C Strategy 2005–2008*. Canberra: Department of Health and Ageing.

Commonwealth of Australia Department of Health and Ageing. 2008. *National Hepatitis C Resource Manual*. Canberra: Department of Health and Ageing.

Conrad, P. and Schneider, A.W. 1980a. *Deviance and Medicalisation: From Badness to Sickness*, 1st edition. St Louis, MO: Mosby.

Conrad, P. and Schneider, A.W. 1980b. Looking at levels of medicalisation: A comment on Strong's critique of the thesis of medical imperialism. *Social Science & Medicine*. 14A, 75-9.

Davis, G. 1999. Hepatitis C virus genotypes and quasispecies. *The American Journal of Medicine*, 107(6B), 21s-6s.

Davis, M. and Rhodes, T. 2004. Managing seen and unseen blood associated with drug injecting: Implications for theorising harm reduction for viral risk. *International Journal of Drug Policy*, 15, 377-84.

Daykin, N. and Naidoo, J. 1995. Feminist Critiques of health promotion, in *The Sociology of Health Promotion: Critical Analyses of Consumption, Lifestyle and Risk*, edited by R. Bunton, S. Nettleton and R. Burrows. London: Routledge, 59-69.

Deleuze, G. 1994. *Difference and Repetition*. London: Athlone Press.

Deleuze, G. and Guattari, F. 1987. *A Thousand Plateaus: Capitalism and Schizophrenia*, translated by Brian Massumi. Minneapolis: University of Minnesota Press.

Derrida, J. 1978. *Writing and Difference*. Chicago: University of Chicago Press.

Dieperink, E., Ho, S.B., Thuras, P. and Willenbring, M.L. 2003. A prospective study of neuropsychiatric symptoms associated with interferon-alpha-2b and ribavirin therapy for patients with chronic hepatitis C. *Psychosomatics*, 44(2), 104-12.

Dieperink, E., Willenbring, M. and Ho, S.B. 2000. Neuropsychiatric symptoms associated with hepatitis C and interferon alpha: A review. *American Journal of Psychiatry*, 157, 867-76.

Dodge, Y. 2003. *The Oxford Dictionary of Statistical Terms*, 6th edition. Oxford: Oxford University Press.

Dolan, M. 1999. *The Hepatitis C Handbook*. Berkeley, CA: North Atlantic Books.

Dowsett, G. 1996. *Practicing Desire: Homosexual Sex in the Era of AIDS.* Stanford: Stanford University Press.

Duffin, J. 2005. *Lovers and Livers: Disease Concepts in History.* Toronto: University of Toronto Press.

Dwyer, R., Fraser, S. and Treloar, C. 2011. Doing things together? Analysis of health promotion materials to inform hepatitis C prevention among couples. *Addiction Research & Theory*, 19(4), 352-61.

Everson, G. and Weinberg, H. 1998, 1999, 2002, 2006. *Living with Hepatitis C: A Survivor's Guide.* New York: Hatherleigh Press.

Forns, X., Bukh, J. and Purcell, R.H. 2002. Review: The challenge of developing a vaccine against hepatitis C virus. *Journal of Hepatology*, 37, 684-95.

Foucault, M. 1973. *The Birth of the Clinic: The Archaeology of Medical Perception.* London: Tavistock.

Foucault, M. 1977/1995. *Discipline and Punish.* Harmondsworth: Penguin.

Foucault, M. 1980a. Body/power, in *Power/knowledge: Selected Interviews and Other Writings 1972–1977*, edited by C. Gordon. New York: Random House, 55-62.

Foucault, M. 1980b. Two lectures, in *Power/knowledge: Selected Interviews and Other Writings 1972–1977*, edited by C. Gordon. New York: Random House, 78-108.

Foucault, M. 1980c. Power and strategies, in *Power/knowledge: Selected Interviews and Other Writings 1972–1977*, edited by C. Gordon. New York: Random House, 134-45.

Foucault, M. 1984. Truth and power, in *The Foucault Reader*, edited by P. Rabinow. New York: Random House, 50-69.

Foucault, M. 1994. The subject and power, in *Essential Works of Foucault 1954–1984, Volume 3: Power*, edited by J.D. Faubion. London: Penguin, 326-48.

Frank, C., Mohamed, M., Strickland, G., Lavanchy, D., Arthur, R., Magder, L., Khoby, T., Abdel-Wahab, Y., Ohn, E. and Anwar, W. 2000. The role of parenteral antischistosomal therapy in the spread of hepatitis C virus in Egypt. *Lancet*, 355(9207), 887-91.

Fraser, N. 1981. Foucault on modern power: Empirical insights and normative confusions. *Praxis International*, 1(3), 272-87.

Fraser, S. 2003. *Cosmetic Surgery, Gender and Culture.* Basingstoke: Palgrave.

Fraser, S. 2004. 'It's Your Life!': Injecting drug users, individual responsibility and hepatitis C prevention. *Health: An Interdisciplinary Journal for the Social Study of Health, Illness and Medicine*, 8(2), 199-221.

Fraser, S. 2011. Beyond the 'potsherd': The role of injecting drug use-related stigma in shaping hepatitis C, in *The Drug Effect: Health, Crime and Society*, edited by S. Fraser and D. Moore. Melbourne: Cambridge University Press.

Fraser, S. and Moore, D. 2011. Harm reduction and hepatitis C: On the ethics and politics of prevention and treatment. *Addiction Research & Theory*.

Fraser, S. and Treloar, C. 2006. 'Spoiled identity' in hepatitis C infection: The binary logic of despair. *Critical Public Health*, 16, 99-110.

Fraser, S. and valentine, k. 2008. *Substance and Substitution: Methadone Subjects in Liberal Societies*. Basingstoke: Palgrave.

Fried, M.W. 2002. Side effects of therapy of hepatitis C and their management. *Hepatology*, 36, S237-S244.

Fried, M.W., Shiffman, M.L., Reddy, K.R., Smith, C., Marinos, G., Goncales, F.L., Häussinger, D., Diago, M., Carosi, G., Dhumeaux, D., Craxi, A., Lin, A., Hoffman, J., Yu, J. 2002. Peginterferon alfa-2a plus ribavirin for chronic hepatitis C virus infection. *New England Journal of Medicine*, 347, 975-82.

Fung, S.K and Lok, A.SF. 2005. Update on viral hepatitis in 2004. *Current Opinion in Gastroenterology*, 21(3), 300-307.

Fyfe, G. and Law, J. 1988. On the invisibility of the visual: Editors' introduction, in *Picturing Power: Visual Depiction and Social Relations*, edited by G. Fyfe and J. Law. London: Routledge, 1-14.

Galvin, R. 2002. Disturbing notions of chronic illness and individual responsibility: Towards a genealogy of morals. *Health: An Interdisciplinary Journal for the Social Study of Health, Illness and Medicine*, 6(2), 107-37.

Goode, E. and Ben-Yehuda, N. 1994. Moral panics: Culture, politics and social construction. *Annual Review of Sociology*, 20, 149-71.

Gutfreund, K.S. and Bain, V.G. 2000. Chronic viral hepatitis C: Management update. *Canadian Medical Association Journal*, 162(6), 827-33.

Hadziyannis, S.J., Sette, H., Morgan, T.R., Balan, V., Diago, M., Marcellin, P., Ramadori, G., Bodenheimer, H., Bernstein, D., Rizzetto, M., Zeuzem, S., Pockros, P.J., Lin, A., Ackrill, A.M. 2004. Peginterferon-alpha2a and ribavirin combination therapy in chronic hepatitis C: a randomized study of treatment duration and ribavirin dose. *Annals of Internal Medicine*, 140, 346-55.

Hall, S. 1996. On Postmodernism and articulation: An interview with Stuart Hall, in *Stuart Hall: Critical Dialogues in Cultural Studies*, edited by D. Morley and K. Chen. London and New York: Routledge, 131-50.

Haraway, D. 1992. The promises of monsters: A regenerative politics for inappropriate/d others, in *Cultural Studies*, edited by L. Grossberg, C. Nelson and P. Treichler. London and New York: Routledge, 295-337.

Harris, M. 2005. Living with hepatitis C: The medical encounter. *New Zealand Sociology*, 20(1), 4-19.

Hartsock, N. 1990. Foucault on power: A theory for women, in *Feminism/ Postmodernism*, edited by L. Nicholson. London: Routledge, 157-73.

Harvey, A.J and Harvey, K.G. 2008. The hazards of blood transfusion in historical perspective. *Blood*, 112(7), 2617-26.

Hazleden, R. 2003. Love yourself: The relationship of the self with itself in popular self-help texts. *Journal of Sociology*, 39(4), 413-28.

Hazleden, R. 2009. Promises of peace and passion: Enthusing the readers of self help. *M/C Journal* [Online], 12(2). Available at: http://journal.media-culture. org.au/index.php/mcjournal/article/view/124 [accessed: 27 January 2011].

Hellard, M., Sacks-Davis, R., Higgs, P. Bharadwaj, M., Bowden, D., Drummer, H. and Aitken, C. 2010. Elispot testing shows very few injecting drug users avoid hepatitis C virus exposure. Poster presented to the International Liver Congress 2010, Vienna, Austria, 14-18 April. Abstract available at: www. kenes.com/easl2010/Posters/Abstract951.htm [accessed: 13 June 2010].

Hepatitis Australia. 2007. *Contact: Post–test Information for Hepatitis C.* ACT: Hepatitis Australia.

Hepatitis C Council NSW. 2009. *Transmission Magazine.* 2nd Edition, June. Darlinghurst: HCC NSW.

Hepatitis C Support Project. 2008. *A Guide to Hepatitis C Treatment Side Effect Management.* [Online: Hepatitis C Support Project]. Available at http://www. hcvadvocate.org/hepatitis/factsheets_pdf/Treatment_Side_effect_Guide.pdf [accessed 13 May 2010].

Hopwood, M. 2009. *Recovery from Hepatitis C Treatments. (Monograph 6/2009).* Sydney: National Centre in HIV Social Research.

Hopwood, M. and Southgate, E. 2003. Living with hepatitis C: A sociological review. *Critical Public Health,* 13(3), 251-67.

Hopwood, M. and Treloar, C. 2003. *The 3-D Project: Diagnosis, Disclosure, Discrimination and Living with Hepatitis C. NCHSR Monograph, No. 6, National Centre in HIV Social Research.* Kensington: University of New South Wales.

Hopwood, M. and Treloar, C. 2005. The experience of interferon-based treatments for hepatitis C infection. *Qualitative Health Research,* 15(5), 635-46.

Hopwood, M. and Treloar, C. 2007. Pretreatment preparation and management of interferon-based therapy for hepatitis C virus infection. *Journal of Advanced Nursing,* 59(3), 248-54.

Hoy, D. 1986. Power, repression, progress: Foucault, Lukes and the Frankfurt School, in *Foucault: A Critical Reader* edited by D.C. Hoy. Oxford: Basil Blackwell, 123-47.

Hughes, C.A and Shafran, S.D. 2006. Chronic hepatitis C virus management: 2000–2005 update. *The Annals of Pharmacotherapy,* 40, 74-82.

Hulse, G. 1997. Australia's public health response to HIV and HCV: A role for 'affected' communities. *Drug and Alcohol Review,* 16, 171-6.

Hunt, C.M., Dominitz, J.A., Bute, B.P. Waters, B., Blasi, U. and Williams, D.M. 1997. Effect of interferon – a treatment of chronic hepatitis C on health-related quality of life. *Digestive Diseases and Sciences.* 42(12), 2482-6.

Hunt, P. and de Luna, W. 2007. *Reading livers through reading literature: HEPATOSCOPY and HARUSPICY in Iliad* [Online]. Available at: http:// traumwerk.stanford.edu/archaeolog/2007/09/reading_livers_through_ reading_1.html [accessed: 11 March 2010].

Hwang, SJ. 2001. Hepatitis C Virus: an overview. *Journal of Microbiological and Immunological Infection*, 34, 227-34.

Illich, I. 1976. *Medical Nemesis*. New York: Pantheon Books.

Keane, H. 2002. *What's Wrong with Addiction?* Carlton South: Melbourne University Press.

Keating, G.M. and Curran, M.P. 2003. Peginterferon alpha-2a (40Kd) plus ribavirin: A review of its use in the management of chronic hepatitis C. *Drugs and Society*, 63(7), 701-30.

Körner, H. 2010. Negotiating treatment for hepatitis C: Interpersonal alignment in the clinical encounter. *Health: An Interdisciplinary Journal for the Social Study of Health, Illness and Medicine*, 14(3), 272-91.

Kraus, M.R., Schaefer, A., Csef, H., Scheurlen, M. and Faller, H. 2000. Emotional state, coping styles and somatic variables in patients with chronic hepatitis C. *Psychosomatics*, 41, 377-84.

Krug, G. 1995. Hepatitis C: Discursive domains and epistemic chasms. *Journal of Contemporary Ethnography*, 24(3), 299-323.

Krug, G. 1997. HCV in the mass media: An unbearable absence of meaning, in *Cultural Studies: A Research Annual. Vol. 2*, edited by N. Denzin. Greenwich, CT and London: Jai Press, 91-108.

Kuhn, T.S. 1957. *The Copernican Revolution. Planetary Astronomy in the Development of Western Thought*. Cambridge, MA: Harvard University Press.

Latour, B. 1987. *Science in Action: How to Follow Scientists and Engineers Through Society*. Milton Keynes: Open University Press.

Latour, B. 2004. Why has critique run out of steam? From matters of fact to matters of concern. *Critical Inquiry*, 30(2), 225-48.

Latour, B. 2005. *Reassembling the Social: An Introduction to Actor-Network Theory*. Oxford: Oxford University Press.

Law, J. 1999. After ANT: Complexity, naming and topology, in *Actor Network Theory and After*, edited by J. Law and J. Hassard. Oxford, UK: Blackwell, 1-14.

Law, J. 2004. *After Method: Mess in Social Science Research*. London and New York: Routledge.

Lenson, D. 1995. *On Drugs*. Minneapolis, MN and London: University of Minnesota Press.

Lenton, E., Fraser, S., Moore, D. and Treloar, C. 2011. Hepatitis C, love and intimacy: Beyond the 'anomalous body'. *Drugs: Education, Prevention and Policy*, 18(3), 228-36.

Leshner, A. 1999. The next generation of drug abuse research. *NIDA Notes* [Online], 14(1). Available at http://www.nida.nih.gov/nida_notes/nnvol14n1/DirRepVol14N1.html [accessed: 16 April 2009].

Levine, H. 1978. The discovery of addiction: Changing conceptions of habitual drunkenness in America. *Journal of Studies on Alcohol*, 39(1), 143-74.

Lindsay, K.L. 1997. Therapy of hepatitis C: Overview. *Hepatology*, 26(3), 71S-7S.

Lupton, D. 1992. Discourse analysis: A new methodology for understanding the ideologies of health and illness. *Australian Journal of Public Health*, 16(2), 145-50.

Lupton, D. 1995. *The Imperative of Health*. London: Sage.

Lupton, D. 1997. Foucault and the medicalisation critique, in *Foucault, Health and Medicine*, edited by A. Petersen and R. Bunton. London and New York: Routledge, 94-110.

Macdonald, G. and Bunton, R. 1992. Health promotion: Disciplinary developments, in *Health Promotion: Disciplines, Diversity, and Developments*, 2nd edition, edited by R. Bunton and G. Macdonald. London: Routledge, 9-27.

Maddrey, W.C. 2001. Update in hepatology. *Annals of Internal Medicine Update Series*, 134, 216-23.

Majer, M., Welberg, L.A., Capuron, L., Pagnoni, G., Raison, C.L., and Miller, A.H. 2008. IFN-alpha-induced motor slowing is associated with increased depression and fatigue in patients with chronic hepatitis C. *Brain, Behavior and Immunity*, 22, 870-80.

Manns, M.P., McHutchison, J.G., Gordon, S.C., Rustgi, V.K., Shiffman, M., Reindollar, R., Goodman, Z.D., Koury, K., Ling, M., Albrecht, J.K. 2001. Peginterferon alfa-2b plus ribavirin compared with interferon alfa-2b plus ribavirin for initial treatment of chronic hepatitis C: A randomised trial. *Lancet*, 358, 958-65.

Martell, M.E.A. 1992. Hepatitis C virus (HCV) circulates as a population of different but closely related genomes: Quasispecies nature of HCV genome distribution. *Journal of Virology*, 66(5), 3225-9.

Más, A., López-Galíndez, C., Cacho, I., Gómez, J. and Martínez, M.A. 2010. Unfinished stories on viral quasispecies and Darwinian views of evolution. *Journal of Molecular Biology*, 397, 865-77.

McHutchison, J.G. and Fried, M.W. 2003. Current therapy for hepatitis C: Pegylated interferon and ribavirin. *Clinics in Liver Disease*, 7(1), 149-61.

McNay, L. 1991. The Foucauldian body and the exclusion of experience. *Hypatia*, 6(3), 125-39.

Mol, A. 1999. Ontological politics: A word and some questions, in *Actor Network Theory and After*, edited by J. Law and J. Hassard. Oxford: Blackwell, 74-89.

Mol, A. 2002. *The Body Multiple: Ontology in Medical Practice*. Durham, NC: Duke University Press.

Mol, A. and Law, J. 2002. Complexities: An introduction, in *Complexities: Social Studies of Knowledge Practices*, edited by J. Law and A. Mol. Durham, NC: Duke University Press, 1-22.

Moore, D. and Fraser, S. 2006. Putting at risk what we know: Reflecting on the drug-using subject in harm reduction and its political implications. *Social Science & Medicine*, 62, 3035-47.

Moradpour, D., Cerny, A., Heim, M.H. and Blum, H.E. 2001. Hepatitis C: An update. *Swiss Medical Weekly*, 131, 291-8.

National Centre in HIV Epidemiology and Clinical Research (NCHECR) 2005. *Annual Surveillance Report: HIV/AIDS, Viral Hepatitis and Sexually Transmitted Infections in Australia.* Sydney: NCHECR, University of NSW.

National Centre in HIV Epidemiology and Clinical Research (NCHECR). 2008a. *HIV/AIDS, Viral Hepatitis and Sexually Transmissible Infections in Australia: Annual Surveillance Report.* Sydney: NCHECR, University of NSW.

National Centre in HIV Epidemiology and Clinical Research (NCHECR) 2008b. *Australian NSP Survey National Data Report 2003–2007.* Sydney: NCHECR, UNSW.

Nettleton, S. 1995. *The Sociology of Health and Illness*, 1st edition. Cambridge: Polity Press.

Nettleton, S. 1996. Women and the new paradigm of health and medicine. *Critical Social Policy*, 16, 33-53.

New South Wales Health. 2008. *Review of Hepatitis C Treatment and Care Services*, New South Wales: NSW Health.

Novas, C. and Rose, N. 2000. Genetic risk and the birth of the somatic individual. *Economy & Society*, 29(4), 485-513.

O'Malley, P., Weir, L. and Shearing, C. 1997. Governmentality, criticism, politics. *Economy and Society*, 26(4), 501-17.

Orsini, M. 2002. The politics of naming, blaming and claiming: HIV, hepatitis C and the emergence of blood tainted activism in Canada. *Canadian Journal of Political Science*, 35(3), 475-98.

Orsini, M. 2008. Hepatitis C and the dawn of biological citizenship: Unravelling the policy implications, in *Contesting Illness: Processes and Practices*, edited by P. Moss and K. Teghtsoonian. Toronto: University of Toronto Press.

Oudshoorn, N. 1994. *Beyond the Natural Body: An Archeology of Sex Hormones.* London: Routledge.

Patterson, B., Backmund, M., Hirsch, G. and Yim, C. 2007. The depiction of stigmatization in research about hepatitis C. *International Journal of Drug Policy*, 18, 364-73.

Patton, P. 1989. Taylor and Foucault on power and freedom. *Political Studies*, 37, 260-76.

Paul, N. 2005. *Living with Hepatitis C for Dummies.* Hoboken, NJ: Wiley.

Pearlman, B.L. 2004a. Hepatitis C infection: A clinical review. *Southern Medical Journal*, 97(4), 365-73.

Pearlman, B.L. 2004b. Hepatitis C treatment update. *American Journal of Medicine*, 117, 344-52.

Pérez, V. 2007. Review article: Viral hepatitis: Historical perspectives from the 20th to the 21st century. *Archives of Medical Research*, 38(6), 593-605

Petersen, A. 1997a. The new morality: Public health and personal conduct, in *Foucault: The Legacy*, edited by C. O'Farrell. Kelvin Grove: Queensland University of Technology, 696-706.

Petersen, A. 1997b. Risk, governance and the new public health, in *Foucault Health and Medicine*, edited by A. Petersen and R. Bunton. London: Routledge, 189-206.

Petersen, A. and Lupton, D. 1996. *The New Public Health: Health and Self in the Age of Risk*. St Leonards: Allen & Unwin.

Plagemann, P. 1991. Hepatitis C virus: Brief review. *Archives of Virology*, 120, 160-80.

Porter, R. 1997. *The Greatest Benefit to Mankind: A Medical History of Humanity*. London: HarperCollins.

Power, C. and Rasko, J.E.J. 2008. Whither Prometheus' liver? Greek myth and the science of regeneration. *Annals of Internal Medicine*, 149, 421-6.

Pugh, J. 2008. Hepatitis C and the Australian news media: A case of 'bad blood'. *Continuum*, 22(3), 385-94.

Purcell, R.H. 1994. Hepatitis viruses: Changing patterns of human disease. *Proceedings of the National Academy of Sciences of the United States of America*, 91(7), 2401-6.

Purcell, R.H. 1997. The hepatitis C virus: Overview. *Hepatology*, 11s-14s.

Purcell, R.H. 2006. Hepatitis C virus: Historical perspective and current concept. *FEMS Microbiology Reviews*, 14(3), 181-91.

Queensland Health. 2005. *Injecting + Infections*. QLD: Exchange Supplies.

Rabinow, P. and Rose, N. 2006. Biopower today. *Biosocieties*, *1*, 195-217.

Raison, C.L., Demetrashvili, M., Capuron, L. and Miller, A.H. 2005. Neuropsychiatric adverse effects of interferon-alpha: Recognition and management. *CNS Drugs*, 19(2), 105-23.

Rhodes, T. and Treloar, C. 2008. The social production of hepatitis C risk among injecting drug users: A qualitative synthesis. *Addiction*, 103, 1593-603.

Ricoeur. P. 1977. *The Rule of Metaphor: Multi-disciplinary Studies of the Creation of Meaning in Language*. Toronto: University of Toronto Press.

Rimke, H. 2000. Governing citizens through self-help literature. *Cultural Studies*, 14(1), 61-78.

Roberts, C., valentine, k. and Fraser, S. 2009. Rationalities and non-rationalities in clinical encounters. *Science as Culture*, 18(2), 165-81.

Rose, N. 1999. *Powers of Freedom: Reframing Political Thought*. Cambridge: Cambridge University Press.

Rose, N. 2007a. *The Politics of Life Itself.* Princeton: Princeton University Press.

Rose, N. 2007b. Beyond medicalisation. *Lancet*. 369(9562), 700-702.

Rosenberg, C.E. 1992. *Explaining Epidemics and Other Studies in the History of Medicine*. Cambridge: Cambridge University Press.

Rosenberg, C.E. 2002. The tyranny of diagnosis: Specific entities an individual experience. *The Milbank Quarterly*, 80(2), 237-60.

Saleh, D.A., Shebl, F.M., El-Kamary, S.S., Magder, L.S., Allam, A., Abdel-Hamid, M., Mikhail, N., Hashem, M., Sharaf, S., Stoszek, S.K. and Strickland, G.T. 2010. Incidence and risk factors for community-acquired hepatitis C infection from birth to 5 years of age in rural Egyptian children. *Transactions of the Royal Society of Tropical Medicine and Hygiene.* 104(5), 357-63.

Sarbah, S.A. and Younossi, Z.M. 2000. Hepatitis C: An update on the silent epidemic, clinical reviews. *Journal of Clinical Gastroenterology*, 30(2), 125-43.

Sarrazin, C. 2004. Diagnosis of hepatitis C: Update 2004. *Journal of Gastroenterology and Hepatology*, 19, S88-S93.

Scott, S. 2006. The medicalisation of shyness: From social misfits to social fitness. *Sociology of Health & Illness.* 28(2), 133-53.

Seddon, T. 2007. Drugs and freedom. *Addiction Research and Theory*, 15(4), 333-42.

Sedgwick, E. 1993. Epidemics of the will, in *Tendencies*, edited by E. Sedgwick. London: Routledge.

Seear, K. 2009a. 'Nobody really knows what it is or how to treat it': Why women with endometriosis do not comply with healthcare advice. *Health, Risk and Society*, 11(4), 367-85.

Seear, K. 2009b. 'Standing up to the beast': Contradictory notions of control, un/certainty and risk in the endometriosis self-help literature. *Critical Public Health*, 19(1), 45-58.

Seear, K. and Fraser, S. 2010. 'The sorry addict': Ben Cousins and the construction of drug use in elite sport. *Health Sociology Review*, 19(2), 176-91.

Seear, K., Fraser, S. and Lenton, E. 2010. Guilty or angry? The politics of emotion in accounts of hepatitis C transmission. *Contemporary Drug Problems*, 37(4), 619-38 .

Sharara, A.I., Hunt, C.M. and Hamilton, J.D. 1996. Update: Hepatitis C. *Annals of Internal Medicine*, 125, 658-68.

Shepard, C., Finelli, L. and Alter, M. 2005. Global epidemiology of hepatitis C virus infection. *Lancet Infectious Diseases*, 5, 558-67.

Sherlock, S. 1996. Hepatitis C virus: A historical perspective. *Digestive Diseases and Sciences*, 41(12), 3S-5S.

Smith, B.C., Strasser, S.I. and Desmond, P.V. 1995. Current perspectives in hepatitis C. *Australian and New Zealand Journal of Medicine*, 25, 350-57.

St John, T. and Sandt, L. 2005. The hepatitis C crisis. *Ethnicity and Disease*, 15(S2), 52-7.

Star, S.L. 1991. Power, technology and the phenomenology of conventions: On being allergic to onions, in *A Sociology of Monsters: Essays on Power, Technology and Domination*, edited by J. Law. London: Routledge, 26-56.

Stenson, K. 1998. Beyond histories of the present. *Economy and Society*, 27(4), 333-52.

Stoové, M.A., Gifford, S.M. and Dore, G.J. 2005. The impact of injecting drug use status on hepatitis C-related referral and treatment. *Drug and Alcohol Dependence*, 77, 81-6.

Tacconelli, E. 2009. *Living Confidently with HIV*. Gloucester: Blue Stallion Publications.

Tatchell, P. 1997. *Fighting Back Against HIV*. London and New York: Continuum.

Taylor, C. 1984. Foucault on freedom and truth. *Political Theory*, 12(2), 152-83.

Tomes, N. 2007. Patient empowerment and the dilemmas of late-modern medicalisation. *Lancet*, 369(9562), 698-700.

Treichler, P. 1999. *How to Have Theory in an Epidemic: Cultural Chronicles of AIDS*. Durham, NC: Duke University Press.

Treloar, C. and Fraser, S. 2004. Hepatitis C, blood and models of the body: New directions for public health. *Critical Public Health*, 14, 377-89.

Treloar, C. and Rhodes, T. 2009. The lived experience of hepatitis C and its treatment among injecting drug users: Qualitative synthesis. *Qualitative Health Research*, 19(9), 1321-34.

Turner, B.S. 1995. *Medical Power and Social Knowledge*, 2nd edition. London: Sage.

Valverde, M. 1998. *Diseases of the Will: Alcohol and the Dilemmas of Freedom*, Cambridge: Cambridge University Press.

Vickerman, P., Miners, A. and Williams, J. 2008. *Assessing the Cost-effectiveness of Interventions Linked to Needle and Syringe Programmes for Injecting Drug Users: An Economic Modeling Report*. London: National Institute for Health and Clinical Excellence.

Victorian Government Department of Human and Community Services. 1995. *Hepatitis C: The Facts*. Melbourne: Health and Community Services Promotion Unit.

Victorian Government Department of Human and Community Services. 1996. *Hepatitis C: The Facts*. Melbourne: Infectious Disease Unit.

Volk, M.L., Tocco, R., Saini, S. and Lok, A.S.F. 2009. Public health impact of antiviral therapy for hepatitis C in the United States, *Hepatology*, 50(6), 1750-55.

Waldby, C. 1996. *AIDS and the Body Politic: Biomedicine and Sexual Difference*. London: Routledge.

Walker, M.A. 1999. Hepatitis C virus: an overview of current approaches and progress. *Drug Discovery Today*, 4(11), 518-29.

Walker, M.P., Appleby, T.C., Zhong, W., Lau, J.Y. and Hong, Z. 2003. Review: Hepatitis C virus therapies: Current treatments, targets and future perspectives. *Antiviral Chemistry & Chemotherapy*, 14, 1-21.

Walsh, K. and Alexander, G.J.M. 2001. Update on chronic viral hepatitis. *Postgraduate Medicine*, 77, 498-505.

Washington, H. 2000. *Living Healthy with Hepatitis C*. New York: Random House.

West, R. 2001. Theories of addiction. *Addiction*, 96, 3-13.

White, W.L. 1998. *Slaying the Dragon: The History of Addiction Treatment and Recovery in America*. Bloomington: Chestnut Health Systems.

White, W.L. 2001. Addiction disease concept: Advocates and critics. *Counselor*, February.

Woerz, I., Lohmann, V. and Bartenschlager, R. 2009. Review: Hepatitis C virus replicons: Dinosaurs still in business? *Journal of Viral Hepatitis*, 16, 1-9.

Wong, W. and Terrault, N. 2005. Reviews: Update on chronic hepatitis C. *Clinical Gastroenterology and Hepatology*, 3, 507-20.

Yu, M.L., Dai, C.Y., Lin, Z.Y., Lee, L.P., Hou, N.J., Hsieh, M.Y., Chen, S.C., Hsieh, M.Y., Wang, L.Y., Chang, W.Y. and Chuang, W.L. 2006. A randomized trial of 24-vs. 48-week courses of PEG interferon alpha-2b plus ribavirin for genotype-1b-infected chronic hepatitis C patients: A pilot study in Taiwan. *Liver International*, 26(1), 73-81.

Zickmund, S., Bryce, C., Blasiole, J., Shinkunas, L., LaBrecque, D. and Arnold, R. 2006. Majority of patients with hepatitis C express physical, mental, and social difficulties with antiviral treatment. *European Journal of Gastroenterology and Hepatology*, 18(4), 381-8.

Zola, I.K. 1972. Medicine as an institution of social control. *Sociological Review*, 20, 487-504.

Zou, S., Forrester, L. and Giulivi, A. 2003. Hepatitis C update. *Canadian Journal of Public Health*, 94(2), 127-9.

Index

Harris, M. 9, 55
HCV (hepatitis C virus) and quasispecies
    epistemology 21-5, 26-9
health promotion
    absence of representative case 52-3
    act of naming 52
    conclusions 61-3
    introduction 41-4
    more than one and less than many
      44-7
    Prometheus' liver 59-61
    virus
      multiple 44, 47-51
      singular 44, 51-2, 53-9
Hepatitis C Council of New South Wales
    47
hepatitis C virus *see* HCV
heroin
    addiction and treatment of hepatitis
      C 28
    Andy 95
    Guiseppe 95, 99, 101
    Stacey 75
HIV
    Africa 7
    'gay' disease 7-8
    hepatitis C
      comparison 68-9, 71
      differences 2
      self-help books 69, 71
    key issues 4
    treatment 7
Hopwood, Max 131
How to Have Theory in an Epidemic:
    Cultural Chronicles of AIDS 6

iatrogenesis 71-2, 75-6, 133, 135
'IDU' populations 11
Illich, Ivan 86, 133-4
injecting drug use (IDU)
    assumptions 31-2
    biological citizenship 83, 84,88, 91
    Bodies that Matter 118
    chemotherapy 116
    combination therapy 136
    community 33
    concept 141
    Ellen 124

Egypt 9
female figure 56
Guiseppe 98, 102, 105
'harms' 117
health promotion 55-60
hepatitis C 1-5, 44, 48, 50, 55, 58,
    134, 141
HIV 7
liver problems 31
Long 127
Lucinda 135
medicalisation benefits 106
people characteristics 125
politics 137
risk 117
self-help literature 65-81
virus threat 60
what is it? 144
see also stigma
Inquiry into Blood Supply and Hepatitis C
    in Australia 72
interferon and ribavarin treatment 27, 131
introduction to hepatitis C 1-3

Journal of Molecular Biology, 2010 20-21
Journal of Virology, 1992 20

Kant, Immanuel 93, 109
Keane, Helen 134
knowing, doing, hoping: limits of
    biological citizenship
    Andy 94-6, 99, 102, 105
    background 85-6
    conclusions: what may we hope?
      108-9
    critique of medicalisation background
      86-8
    Guiseppe 94, 96-9, 101-2, 105-7
    introduction 83-4
    Kant's three questions 93, 109
    from medicalisation to biological
      citizenship? 92-3
    medicalising addiction 88-92
    Stacey 94, 99-104
    what can I know, what must I do? 94

Lalonde, Marc 42
Lalonde Report 42

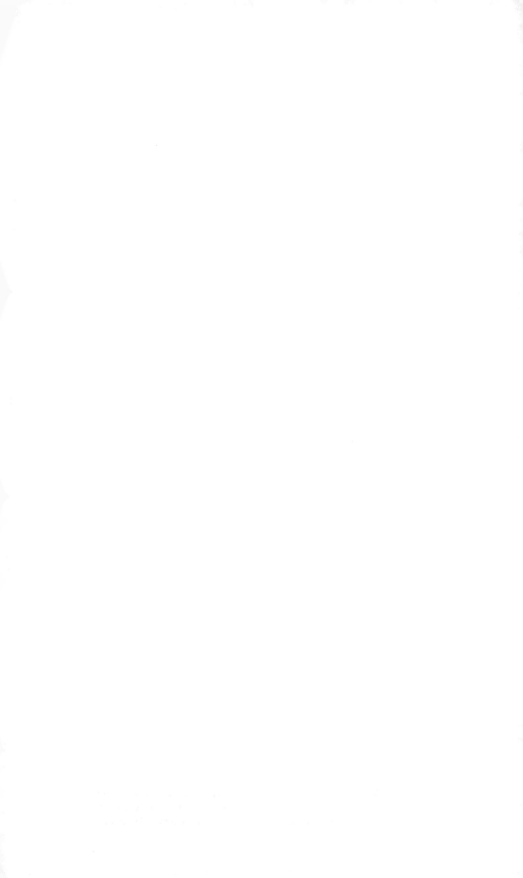